Medical Dissertations of Psychiatric Interest
Printed before 1750

Medical Dissertations of Psychiatric Interest

Printed before 1750

OSKAR DIETHELM
Prof. em. of psychiatry
Cornell University Medical College, New York

S. Karger · Basel · München · Paris · London · New York · Sydney · 1971

This work has been supported in part by a research grant from the USPHS (National Institute of Mental Health).

S. Karger · Basel · München · Paris · London · New York · Sydney
Arnold-Böcklin-Strasse 25, CH–4000 Basel 11 (Switzerland)

Contents

Preface

A clinician and teacher is under obligation to study current and past medical literature, thus increasing his knowledge and widening his critical perspective.

History of medicine was frequently taught as if the growth and development of psychiatry was essentially limited to the last two centuries and its connection to psychology, philosophy and cultural changes was neglected. The relationship to medicine in general was recognized but historically little explored.

In the period of 1925 to 1935 when I was at the Johns Hopkins Medical School, under the leadership of ADOLF MEYER psychiatric practice and teaching had become part of medicine. FREUD's contribution became increasingly evaluated. The development of the Department of History of Medicine forced the clinician to look for a better orientation in his special field. With this background, I considered it an essential task to develop a historical psychiatric library at Cornell University Medical College when I joined the faculty in 1936. At that time I found nowhere a library which could offer a satisfactory collection of books for a historical orientation in psychiatry. With the growth of the library we became increasingly aware of the lack of well-established psychiatric data in various periods of medical history. Every effort was made to gather good descriptions of clinical material, containing sufficient details to illustrate the gradual development of theories and practice. Observations, published since the 16th century, offered an opportunity to fill to some extent the gaps in the development of psychiatry, indicating that since the Renaissance progress had been greater and more steady than had been assumed. Recognizing the contribution of many medical dissertations of the past and present centuries, those of earlier centuries were collected and studied. The results are presented in this book. The search for these dissertations led to many libraries in this country and abroad.

I wish to take this opportunity to express my gratitude to the many librarians and their staffs who helped me and made me feel welcome.

Professor Thomas F. Heffernan (Adelphi University) wrote the scholarly translations which are included here. Without his valuable contribution it would have been difficult to write this text.

I also wish to acknowledge my appreciation to the Confinia Psychiatrica for permission to reprint the chapter on mania, and to the Journal of the History of the Behavioral Sciences. From time to time I have quoted without specification material from a paper *Felix Platter and Psychiatry,* J. Hist. behav. Sci. *1:* 10–23 (1965).

Introduction

The leading textbooks of medicine at the beginning of the 17th century display a considerable interest in psychiatric disorders. The ancient authorities, GALEN and AVICENNA, are still held in high regard, but there is a turning away from them. Instead, there is an increasing number of references to observations, especially those of FORESTUS. But there is no critical analysis. As the 17th and then the 18th centuries passed, books contained more and more observations, as did the developing medical journals.

As the survey that led to this book progressed, it soon became obvious that a few dissertations of the 17th and early 18th centuries contained satisfactory descriptions of cases while others simply offered a detailed review of literature. It was, therefore, decided to establish what case material could be found, how the patients corresponded to our current clinical knowledge, and what differences could be observed in the clinical picture during the last four centuries. A review of the literature at various periods, it was hoped, would increase our understanding of the change in theories and treatment. An evaluation of the dissertations as an educational tool and a clarification of the place of psychiatry in medical education were also planned.

Our conclusion is that the dissertations offer much information about the status of psychiatry in various periods and in different localities. They apprise us of the degree of influence of well-known authors and help to clarify their place in medicine and especially psychiatry. Sometimes an author whose name is now barely known but who is shown to have had some limited influence is quoted. There is little advance noted in treatment, but the varying emphasis on certain aspects reveals attitudes current at the time.

Many teachers in the period of this study had devoted much of their time to anatomical investigations and work in laboratories. The resulting scientific attitude affected their clinical experience, and they demanded accurate observations from their students. But in psychiatry, theories were usually not available to account for many findings. Enthusiasm for the brilliant teacher's theoretical conclusions resulted in the formation of schools with uncritical rigidity. A striking example is found in the dissertations carried out under the direction of FRIEDRICH HOFFMANN and GEORG ERNST STAHL. These teachers' theories of the mind-body relationship were quite divergent, and each attracted a strong group of followers.

A more valuable result is demonstrated by professors who gave the same topic to two or more students during a period of several years.

Diagnostic discussions are stressed in most of the dissertations. They attempt critical evaluations of both the students' observations and of the available literature.

The dissertations tell us little about how people actually lived, about the stresses of daily life and the social problems. Except for an interest in suicide, psychiatry kept separate from the progress of public health. We know from other sources that in general the health and economic security of the student were unsatisfactory and sometimes most deplorable. The housing and food were inadequate, since many of the students came from poor families. Social life and recreation were limited. Student alcoholism was a severe health problem, largely minimized or disregarded by the teachers. In some German universities the professor's own drinking interfered with his professional duties, but this seems to have been tolerated. University administrations had difficulty in controlling the deportment of the students, but it is not possible to determine to what extent medical students contributed to such problems.

The students were privileged to change to other medical schools whenever and as often as they desired, to choose lectures and courses, and to prolong their studies indefinitely. This freedom, which had many educational advantages, presented a serious hazard to the emotional unstable, poorly motivated and immature student. It cannot be stated how many of these students were psychopathologically sick or were not able to finish their studies for economic reasons. The expenses for obtaining a doctoral degree were high, and no doubt many good students had to be satisfied with the baccalaureate.

Despite the well-recognized contribution to legal medicine, including psychiatry, by ZACCHIAS [1657], further interest in this subject did not develop until the end of the 17th century. The dissertations in the 18th century reviewed cases of homicide, especially infanticide, and suicide, but only in the 19th century did alcoholic and sexual problems, including rape, become the concern of physicians and psychiatrists.

The topics for dissertations were usually well selected, illustrating the problems which were in need of clarification.

Yet some of the questions put to the students by the medical faculty of Paris might be considered ridiculous. A study of the psychiatric questions, however, reveals that they deal with problems which were of importance to the physicians. Put in modern medical language, some of these questions still cannot be answered satisfactorily. A question repeated after a hundred years demonstrates the slow progress of medicine and the need for teachers to re-evaluate, with increased knowledge having become available, the answers which had been previously found acceptable.

Dissertations contributed to the increase of psychiatric knowledge by the description of clinical observation, done at considerable length and with accurate detail, its analysis and its correlation to past and current literature. In some dissertations one finds a more detailed account of the psychological approach to the patient than in textbooks and medical treatises. Others illustrate the gradual development of psychotherapy by use of reassurance, suggestion, and an attempt at analysis of life situations.

The teaching value of dissertations was regarded highly. While the presentation of theses in the scholastic form was rejected as a mere exercise in logic, the dissertation forced the students to carry out anatomical, laboratory or clinical observations, to evaluate them critically, and to present them in a well-written form. One is impressed by the interest which some of the professors took in their students. When the instructors became too much interested in a lucrative practice and spent insufficient time in teaching, many medical schools deteriorated.

In some universities monthly or less frequent disputations and exercitia were valuable methods of medical education. They did not differ fundamentally from our modern seminars.

The study of psychiatric dissertations illuminates somewhat the changing relationship of the medical faculty to the university. In psychiatry, the physician is confronted with the patients' problems, including philosophical, legal and cultural implications. The scientific development affected the research and teaching of medicine, but a close relationship between science and humanities was maintained during the period discussed. The dominance of the humanities gradually diminished, but the great scientific investigators and teachers in medicine possessed a broad humanistic background and revealed an understanding of philosophy. This awareness became less obvious in the 19th century. With the growth of teaching hospitals, laboratories and scientific institutes, medical faculties and universities moved further apart. This trend accelerated in the 20th century with the development of medical centers which were often physically removed from the university. In some countries, independent medical schools with mere peripheral contact with a university have been promoted. These became essentially technical schools.

Chapter I
The Rise of Universities and Medical Education

The universities, with legally established independence and freedom of teaching, evolved in the beginning of the 13th century from the learning and teaching in the monasteries and cathedral schools[1,2]. Paris and Bologna, and soon afterwards Oxford, became centers of learning, with faculties of theology, law, medicine and philosophy (including liberal arts). The university was open to students of all nationalities. The many universities which developed during the 14th and 15th centuries were well-supported by the governments of princes and cities, and teachers were held in high esteem.

The Italian Universities which developed in the 14th century attracted students to their medical schools from Northern countries up to the end of the 16th century. Students were grouped, without discrimination, according to the nationalities. A sound rivalry developed between the universities of Bologna, Ferrara, Padua, Pavia and Pisa, with professors and students transferring readily from one university to another. Universities developed in Germany in the 14th and 15th centuries[3]. An interchange of teachers made for some competition and improved standards of teaching. New universities appointed promising young men who had been taught in leading centers by outstanding teachers.

The tendency on the part of various governments to interfere with the universities was not always easy to overcome. Prague (founded in 1355) was the first university which stressed national and political-religious aspects which led to the exodus of German professors and students (1409) to Leipzig where a university was founded. In Spain, the univer-

---

1   D'IRSAY, op. cit.
2   RASHDALL, op. cit.
3   The year of the foundation of a university does not always coincide with the establishing of a medical faculty. Avignon, founded in 1303, had no medical school until the end of the 16th century. (V. LAVAL, Histoire de la faculté de médecine d'Avignon, Paris et Avignon 1889.) Altdorf (1577) started medical education in 1622, Strasbourg (1566) in 1621.

sities of Salamanca (1243), and Valladolid (1346) flourished, absorbing Arabic cultural influences. An increasing domination by state and church became noticeable in the 14th and 15th centuries, and led to full control in the 16th century. In Portugal medical studies flourished during the Renaissance but, after the expulsion of Jewish physicians and domination by the Catholic Church, there was a rapid decline which was aggravated during the Spanish rule (1580 to 1640)[4].

In France, the influence of the university of Paris, which followed scholastic teaching, was challenged by that of Montpellier. This university, founded in the 13th century, was greatly affected by Arabian culture and in the 15th century by the influx of Jewish teachers who had to leave Spain. The danger of persecution for hereticism, which was marked in the South of France[5], must have, however, restricted freedom of teaching.

With the Renaissance, the rejection of dogmatism and the rigidity of scholastic thinking was followed by freedom of thinking and teaching which is clearly seen in some of the Italian and Northern universities[6]. The humanistic atmosphere in the city of Basel permitted the small university which was founded in 1460 to flourish. When freed of Spanish rule, Holland was able to develop its universities (Leyden 1575, Utrecht 1634). German humanism became the strong factor in revitalizing the old and in stimulating the creation of new universities[7]. Infringement of teaching and learning was rejected. Whenever a government or church power succeeded in intruding, professors and students began to leave and the university declined. An interesting example is presented by the flourishing university of Tübingen which, during the Thirty Years' War, came under the control of the Jesuits. The medical school declined rapidly. Even at the time of ALBRECHT HALLER (1725) who had enrolled as a medical student, anatomy was taught by dissection of dogs. HALLER

4   The decline of the Spanish and Portuguese medical faculties is demonstrated by the lack of publications contributing to the development of medicine during the 17th and 18th centuries (GRANJEL, op. cit.).

5   F. PLATTER, Autobiographie (English translation: Beloved son Felix, London 1961).

6   Publications from the medical faculties of Northern Italy, Basel and Tübingen offer outstanding examples of this change.

7   The universities of Basel and Holland became centers of humanism while Louvain and Würzburg were under the influence of Jesuits. The scholastic Aristotelian influence remained important in Frankfurt a. O., Greifswald and Rostock (H. HAESER, op. cit., vol. II, pp. 4–5).

changed to Leyden to study anatomy[8]. Heidelberg was another medical school which suffered similarly[9]. In other German cities where there were universities, if there were a change from a Catholic to a Protestant government, or vice versa, the medical school might have been affected temporarily. Religious difficulties between Lutherans and Calvinists hampered the development of Giessen and Wittenberg[10]. The universities of countries with centralized governmental administrations (France, Portugal and Spain) became influenced or ruled by governmental policies and edicts as early as in the 16th century[11]. The decline in Portugal and Spain relates to restrictions imposed on the cultural development in the 16th and 17th centuries[12], including the acquisition of knowledge from universities outside these kingdoms[13].

The great plagues, wars and periods of famine frequently interfered with the functioning of universities and led to their temporary or permanent closing[14]. In the beginning of the 17th century, Tübingen had to be temporarily transferred to cities which were free of the plague while Giessen was closed for several months (1613). Physical destruction led to the moving of the faculty and students to another university, e.g., Rostock to Greifswald or Marburg to Giessen. Such difficulties did not end in disaster because the faculty could be kept intact.

Teaching in the medical schools changed greatly during the end of the 15th century. Scholastic education was based on reading from the

8   HENRY E. SIGERIST, *Albrecht von Haller,* Grosse Schweizer, Zürich 1938, p. 251.

9   E. STÜBLER, *Geschichte der medizinischen Fakultät der Universität Heidelberg,* Heidelberg 1926.

10   BECKER, *op. cit.* and H. KILIAN, *Die Universitäten Deutschlands in medizinisch-naturwissenschaftlicher Hinsicht,* Heidelberg and Leipzig 1828.

11   DELAUNAY, *op. cit.*

12   FRIEDENWALD, *op. cit.,* documents the loss of Jewish physicians to Spain and Portugal and its resulting gain to universities of Southern France and Italy.

13   The organization of the universities and the ineffective efforts at corrections of increasing academic difficulties by PHILIPPE II and PHILIPPE III are discussed by MARCELIN DEFOURNEAUX, *La vie quotidienne en Espagne au siècle d'or,* Paris 1964, pp. 190–195.

14   The effect of those catastrophies is summarized by HIRSCH, *op. cit.,* p. 80 and given in details in the publication of STÜBLER, *op. cit.* and BECKER, *op. cit.* who illustrates the struggle of a small university in Northern Germany. French universities suffered less from wars but were affected by epidemics of plague (DELAUNAY, *op. cit.* p. 34). Political changes had a limited influence on medical teaching at Strasbourg, a German city which in 1681 became part of France, Dissertations were continued and no coercion seems to have been exerted to accept the French system of theses.

books of GALEN and AVICENNA, with reference to ARISTOTLE, and interpretations by the reader (professor). The student was required to explain
the authors and to defend his answers in the prescribed logical form. In
the 15th and 16th centuries, the reading from great authors (the lectures
of the preceding period) and the strict acceptance of their statements
changed into discussions with independent interpretations. The demon-
stration of dissections and pathological findings resulted in a questioning
and searching attitude by teachers and students. Surgical procedures
were demonstrated and the advanced student was invited to accompany
the professor on his visits to patients. Botanical gardens were developed
to acquaint the students with the herbs recommended for treatment.

The examination for the degree of physician (baccalaureate or master's degree) and license to practice, and especially for the high degree
of doctor of medicine, included a knowledge of the literature of the
Greek, Roman and Arabic, and, increasingly, recent authors[15]. In addition, the student was examined in anatomy, botany, and clinical medicine. In the 17th century, chemistry and physics became important
fields. Physiology began to equal anatomy in its place in the medical
teaching of the 18th century, and public health and legal medicine received attention.

In German universities the teaching of surgery and obstetrics[16] was
included in medical schools, and dissertations from these fields were frequent.

The degree of doctor of medicine, which could only be given by a
university, was the sign of outstanding knowledge of a physician, indicating that he was a scholar and qualified to be a teacher[17]. In some
countries, with several small universities which had a limited medical
faculty, students could obtain only the baccalaureate. In France and
Spain several universities were thus restricted[18]. In Switzerland, Zurich

15 BECKER, *op. cit.* and HIRSCH, *op. cit.*

16 Surgery was taught by the professor of anatomy but inadequately until the
18th century (T. H. BAAS, *Die geschichtliche Entwicklung des ärztlichen Standes
und der medizinischen Wissenschaften,* Berlin 1896).

17 ALBRECHT BURCKHARDT, *op. cit.* discusses the changes during the period from
1466 to 1900, including curriculum and examinations.

18 Most French (DELAUNAY, *op. cit.*) and Spanish universities had inadequate
medical faculties and a small number of students. In the 17th century and especially at the end of the 18th and the beginning of the 19th centuries the governments of France, Germany and Holland closed several of these universities or
combined them with others.

and Schaffhausen offered good practical education but, as these schools were not connected with a university, no degree of doctor could be conferred. English physicians obtained their degree from universities of Northern Italy and after the reformation from Dutch universities[19]. The relatively small number of doctors were greatly honored. In some countries they were ennobled and received the privileges of noblemen. More important, a doctorate offered a career in the academic field, an opportunity to become the physician in attendance at the court of a prince of the world or of the church, or the leading physician of a city. Such a senior physician, with the title of archiater, was elected to maintain high standards among the physicians in the city, to supervise the hospitals and to advise the political authorities with regard to public health. In Basel, when PLATTER was professor and archiater he was requested to be accompanied by students on his (irregular) visits to the city's six hospitals[20].

The election of professors[21] became corrupted in many medical schools through nepotism or actual bribery. A royal edict in France in 1540 tried unsuccessfully to abolish these practices. Election on merit with a publicly announced competition became the custom in the 17th century and was requested in France in 1689. (The title of such a thesis was 'pro vacante sede medica'[22].)

Psychiatric teaching was limited to a discussion of pertinent passages by prominent Greek, Arabic, and Renaissance authors. In the 16th century the text-books paid increasing attention to the presentation of current and past theories but contained little detailed case material. The student's attention was directed to the observations and, to a lesser degree, consultations of the outstanding French, Italian, German and Dutch authors. The student was induced to consider critically what was observed by others or himself and not merely to accept a statement on authority.

19   R. W. INNES-SMITH, *English speaking students of medicine at the University of Leyden,* Edinburgh 1932.
20   Active clinical teaching was started in Leyden by HEURNE (early 17th century) and developed by DE LE BOË (SYLVIUS) and BOERHAAVE.
21   Nomination of a new professor was made by the members of the faculty and usually accepted by the government. Abuses lead frequently to increased control by the government.
22   Several printed contributions by candidates are mentioned by HUSNER, *op. cit.,* p. 12. The titles were thesis, specimen, observations.

Dissertations have gone through a long evolution. The medieval universities, following a scholastic teaching, required the presentation of a thesis. The student discussed the question ('quaestio') which the professor put to him from the point of view of authorities in the field. The answer was presented by the student in five paragraphs. The first paragraph elucidated the question in relation to definition and literature. The second paragraph presented points in favor of an affirmative answer, the third those leading to a negative answer. The fourth paragraph gave an enumeration of the symptoms, the fifth their analysis in relation to the question. Finally, the student's logical conclusion was presented in one sentence, rephrasing the question into an affirmative, rarely a negative, answer. It appears that the presiding professor formulated the question but there are no indications that he influenced the student otherwise[23]. Paris and Reims used this classical form of theses, while in Montpellier the student had more freedom in answering the question[24]. In Spain and Portugal the scholastic form persisted[25].

With the development of scientific medicine in the 16th century, theses were replaced by dissertations[26]. The teachers of Renaissance medicine rejected the blind following of the great physicians of the past and requested the observation of facts, their investigation, and when possible, experimental proof. The acceptance of doctrines was replaced by questioning. This procedure became a well-established teaching tool. The students participated in disputations called 'exercitii gratia' which

---

23   The French educational system is discussed by LEGRAND *(op. cit.),* DELAUNAY *(op. cit.)* and OCTAVE GUELLIOT, *Les thèses de l'Ancienne Faculté de Médecine de Reims,* Reims 1889.

24   In the 18th century professors in French medical schools protested that theses were a futile exercise in logic (LE FRANÇOIS, *Dissertations contre l'usage de soutenir des thèses en médecine,* Paris 1720. The submission of requests to the parliament for changes in teaching met with no response. Reorganization occurred with the French revolution when medical education became organized (LEGRAND, *op. cit.*).

25   Theses were not printed in Portugal and Spain and manuscripts were not available to me at Salamanca and Valladolid. At Coimbra theses are kept in bound volumes. They were brief and in summarized style. Psychiatric topics were rare. There were some discussions of hysteria, phrenitis, catalepsy, melancholia and disorders of memory. Reading them one wonders occasionally whether the author reviewed the literature, or merely abstracted, or put in free translation passages from Greek and Arabic authors.

26   The correct term for a dissertation for the degree of doctor was 'dissertatio inauguralis', inauguralis indicating the ceremonial installation to the office.

were held at stated intervals – biweekly, monthly, or bimonthly[27]. The requirements varied in the different universities. Montpellier, e.g., requested three disputations before a student was permitted to present a dissertation. Usually disputations were not printed, but the more interesting discussions under well-known professors have found a place in medical literature[28]. Until the early part of the 17th century, monthly disputations included frequently two or more respondents. At times each respondent gave his own presentation which appeared in print.

The dissertation was written like a treatise with considerable freedom in form and length. According to the interest of the professor the topic might be from anatomy, physiology, therapeutics or clinical medicine. The student might deal with the topic by presenting his own investigations of clinical case material, or by discussing theoretical aspects. Although the form of the dissertation varied, there was always a review of pertinent literature, a presentation of the student's own observations, a discussion of them and, finally, the conclusions[29].

27 I found in literature no detailed review of exercitia. For an understanding of their value one must turn to printed exercitia (some are listed in HUSNER, *op. cit.* or to the collections of HORST, TANDLER and KNOBLOCH *(op.cit.).*
28 HUSNER, *op. cit.*
29 The progress of medicine and its teaching was lead during the 17th and 18th centuries by the teachers in England, France, Germany and Holland. A valuable contribution to an understanding of the difficulties in France was written by MAURICE RAYNAUD, *Les médecins au temps de Molière,* Paris 1863.

Chapter II
Psychiatric Knowledge in the History of Medicine

During the period from 1550 to 1750 the teaching of HIPPOCRATES[1] was highly regarded and GALEN and the Arabic philosophers still exerted an important influence in many medical schools. A brief review of the development of medicine and a more detailed discussion of the history of psychiatry will serve as a basis for the succeeding chapters.

Starting with HIPPOCRATES observations and the recording of the manifestations of disease replaced philosophical speculation. Two trends which have, in varying degree, influenced medical thinking and practice became obvious. The one, represented by the school of Knidos, was interested in symptoms and diagnosis and a corresponding stereotyped treatment. The other group, on the island of Kos, under the leadership of HIPPOCRATES, centered its attention on the patient and attempted to study etiology in its broad sense and to determine the essential symptoms. The course of the illness was evaluated in reaching diagnosis, prognosis and treatment. Greek natural philosophy, which attributed diseases to disorders of the fluids of the body, was the basis for the humoral pathology of HIPPOCRATES. He postulated that the four elements of fire, air, earth and water are expressed in the four humors of the body – the warmth of blood originating from the heart, the coldness of mucous from the brain, the dryness of yellow gall from the liver, and the humidity of black gall from the spleen. These humors are balanced in the body and an illness occurs when the balance of the mixture is disturbed. The physician was warned against generalizing and theorizing when dealing with a patient. The guiding principle in treatment was that one is dealing with a sick person with diseased organs. The main emphasis was placed on correct diet and a healthy mode of living, to strengthen nature's efforts at recovery and to assist in the removal of the noxious substances by means of diaphoretics, purgatives and clysters, emetics and bleeding.

1   HIPPOCRATES, *op. cit.*

This teaching ruled, or greatly influenced, medicine from the Hellenic period through the 18th century.

ARISTOTLE's (384–322 B.C.) contribution to biology and his philosophy strengthened the teaching of the Hippocratic school but the danger gradually became obvious that his proposal of using deductive methodology decreased the interest in careful observation. He postulated that ether was the principle of living and that life is expressed in movement. The heart was considered the seat of the soul and the center of the vascular system, the brain was the organ which secretes mucous (phlegm) thus cooling excessive heat in the heart. His psychological formulations dominated medical thinking until the Renaissance.

The teaching of HIPPOCRATES was followed in the medical school of Alexandria (founded in 332 B.C.), which played an important role in bringing this knowledge to Syria and Persia and thus helped in the development of Arabian medicine in the medieval period.

Under the leadership of ASCLEPIADES (124 B.C.) for a brief period humoral pathology was replaced by solidism. On the atomic theory of DEMOCRITOS, it was postulated that the body is formed of solid particles and these have the characteristic of constriction and relaxation. A disorder of tonus results in disease. In a different form this theory was proposed again at the end of the 19th century[2].

Other schools are mentioned and their representatives severely critized by GALEN (129 to ca. 198 A.D.) who returned to the teaching of HIPPOCRATES but who, as an eclectic, developed his own school which dominated medical thinking until the Renaissance period, and still remained an important force in the 17th century. He represented the end of the period of critical observation[3] which was made the basis for conclusions in the method of the Alexandrian school. He used dialectic generalizations and conclusions to build a system of the whole field of medicine which presented a seductive security to the physicians[4]. His extraordinary literary productivity included a broad commentary an HIPPO-

2   JOHN BROWN's theory (Elementa medicina, 1780) affected psychiatric treatment, leading to abuse of opium, alcohol and bleeding. His followers included BENJAMIN RUSH. F. T. V. BROUSSAIS offered a theory which explained disease by localized irritation. His advice to use excessive bleeding and a weakening dietary regime influenced the treatment of psychiatric disorders in France and Germany during the beginning of the 19th century.

3   K. SUDHOFF, Geschichte der Medizin, Berlin 1922, offered this evaluation of GALEN.

4   GALEN, op. cit.

CRATES' aphorism. By emphasis on anatomy and physiology he attempted to offer a scientific basis of medicine but by his philosophical speculations, and guided by teleology, he limited his own scientific curiosity and that of his followers. His humoral pathology accepted the four humors, but postulated that blood, a hot and moist humor, comes from the heart; phlegm (mucous) a cold and moist humor, comes from the brain; yellow bile, a hot and dry humor comes from the liver; black bile, a cold and dry humor, comes from the spleen and stomach. In a state of health the humors are properly mingled, but in different quantities according to the individual temperament which had developed during a person's life but also depends on his constitution. According to the humor which predominates, one distinguishes between sanguine, phlegmatic, choleric and melancholic temperaments[5]. In disease, a defect or irregularity occurs in the mixture[6]. This is called dyscrasia or disharmony. The causes for dyscrasia may be congenital, accidental, or determined by natural phenomena (e.g., weather and climate). Treatment followed Hippocratic teaching, based on the study of the patient, and tried to remove the cause, correct the preponderant and disturbing humor and treat the illness. Every disease has its specific remedy. Qualitative and quantitative differences in medicines were carefully listed. The therapeutic principle of 'contraria contrariis' was closely followed. The use of drugs had increased greatly and the prescriptions of DIOSCORIDES OF ALEXANDRIA were recommended.

GALEN wrote that life is dependent on pneuma, received from the surrounding air and consisting of the spiritus animalis (located in the brain), spiritus vitalis (in heart and arteries, regulating the heat in the body), and spiritus naturalis (in the liver, preparing the blood and directing metabolism). The spirits have attracting, expulsive, digestive and occult (hidden) qualities. The animal spirits direct sensations and movements. The body serves the soul and the various organs are the tools which make it possible for the soul to carry out its functions. The brain is the center of the soul (psychic function).

In his writings GALEN refers to HIPPOCRATES and ARISTOTLE and oc-

---

5   The concept of temperament presents a significant attempt to understand the individual person and the relationship of emotions, behavior and physiological functions. These theories became of importance in the 18th, 19th and 20th centuries.

6   Mental disorders, GALEN postulated, originate in the loss of phlegm from the brain, resulting in the decrease of humidity.

casionally to SORANUS and critically attacks ASCLEPIADES as well as members of the methodist school[7].

Arabic medicine, which blossomed from ca. 800 to 1400, was built on GALEN's teaching[8]. The influence of RHAZES (850–932) can be seen from the use of the *Rhazes ad Almansorem* until the 17th century[9]. The most important textbook was the *Canon of Avicenna* (ALI IBN SINA, 980–1037) which closely followed the books of GALEN. The large volume is well organized and more easily read than GALEN. It was soon accepted blindly and followed rigidly during the remainder of the medieval period.

CONSTANTINUS AFRICANUS (ca. 1020–1087) translated Arabian writers into Latin and thus also offered an understanding of Greek medicine including parts of HIPPOCRATES and GALEN. In the 13th and 14th centuries medical teachers in the universities of Italy and of Montpellier began to review older authors instead of merely following the accepted Arabic authorities[10]. They made their own contributions in their textbooks and reviewed case material in consilia. Medicine had entered a stage where dogmatism was questioned, and a need for personal observation and corroboration or new conclusions began to come to the surface in books and in teaching.

History of Psychiatry

The leaders who had a permanent influence on the teaching of medicine before the 16th century were HIPPOCRATES, GALEN and AVICENNA[11]. Their references to psychiatric problems were quoted in the books of the medical teachers of the 15th and 16th centuries. Much of the

7   These authors and those of the Byzantine period which played a role in psychiatric history will be discussed later.

8   Arabic culture in Spain was affected by the past development of the country since the Roman occupation (J. B. TRENT, *op. cit.*) and resulted in a Moorish culture which showed marked Western influences (DIEPGEN, *op. cit.*, vol. I, p. 179).

9   The compendium, like *Rhazes ad Almansorum* is complete while his large comprehensive work, *Continens* is only known in parts. The most quoted book is the 9th (nonus ad Almansorum).

10   Among these critical authors might be mentioned ARNALD OF VILLANOVA (†1311) and ANTONIO GUAINERIO (†1440).

11   FALK (*op. cit.*) wrote an outstanding study of the psychiatric literature before the Arabic period.

teaching consisted of the professor's reading and interpreting the books of GALEN and AVICENNA.

HIPPOCRATES' important contribution to psychiatry was his attention to the patient as an individual and to his physical and psychological needs. He demonstrated the importance of writing down one's observations, of grouping symptoms and of noting changes during the progress of the illness. His aphorisms present conclusions in a concise form, often to such an extent that some meanings remain unclear. They deal primarily with delirious illnesses and refer only infrequently to mania and melancholia. Until the 18th century they were frequently quoted to support some special treatment of psychiatric disorders, e.g., the importance of the free flow of hemorrhoids and menstruation, of discharge from the nose, of excretion of the urine and of bowel movements[12]. His observations offer good descriptions of deliria of an infectious nature. The contributory factors mentioned are excessive consumption of alcohol and insufficient discharge of lochia (indicating puerperal psychosis). The various symptoms which may occur during the course of a delirium are mentioned, e.g., fear, depression or elation, anger, incoherent speech and confusion, periods of silence and food refusal and the inability to remember in lucid intervals experiences occurring during an intense phase. In another book[13] he attacks the belief that divine influence causes incubus, somnambulism and psychiatric illnesses.

It is difficult to evaluate his descriptions and to compare them to illnesses described in modern psychiatry. A statement, not elucidated by other discussion, seems to summarize his general psychiatric attitude:

'If the brain is corrupted by phlegm the patients are quiet and silent; if by bile, they are vociferous, malignant and act improperly. If the brain is heated, terrors, fears and terrifying dreams occur; if it is too cool the patients are grieved and troubled.'[14]

The treatment follows his general principles. The discussion of the diet and mode of living reveals his sympathy and an open-minded attitude.

12   In the *Book of the Epidemics* HIPPOCRATES offers his observations of post-partum psychoses (cases II and XIV in book III), deliria (cases IV, XIII, XV and XVI in book I), melancholia case XI, book III) and of impotence (book IV).
13   *The Sacred Disease* illustrates HIPPOCRATES' broad clinical knowledge, including somnambulism, incubus and psychiatric illnesses, and his psychological understanding of the patient. The *Aphorisms* offer brief statements on delirium, mania and melancholia.
14   HIPPOCRATES, *op. cit.,* The sacred disease.

The psychiatric contribution of ASCLEPIADES is difficult to evaluate. He was seldom quoted until the reference to his writings by CAELIUS AURELIANUS (5th C. A.D.)[15]. It is difficult to determine what his psychiatric observations and attitudes were and what belongs to the editor (CAELIUS AURELIANUS) or SORANUS. ASCLEPIADES defined mental impairment as 'an affection in the senses' which occurs through stoppage of the corpuscules in the membranes of the brain. When the disease is chronic and without fever it is mania (furor); when acute, with fever and without feeling, it is delirium (phrenitis). Among the causes are mentioned hot weather, seasonal changes, the temperament of the patient and his age.

Opposed to the dogmatic school, SORANUS EPHESIUS (98–138 A.D.) stressed the importance of careful observation and evaluation of all the symptoms. The acute diseases, with or without fever, include delirium. Mental aberration may become noticeable before or after the fever period and are recognized by unusually quiet behavior or loud laughter, singing or sadness, muttering, rage or fear. Hallucinations are stressed, expressed in talking to the dead and movements of the hands before the eyes as if to remove objects flying before them. He differentiated between delirium, mania and melancholia. Delirium occurs in febrile disease and from drugs. In the course of mania fever, which is not related to the cause of the mental illness, may occur. In delirium fever comes first, in mania loss of reason is the first sign. In children with fever SORANUS observed attacks which might have been cataleptic or hysterical symptoms. He postulated that laughter and dancing in a delirium is caused by stricture. Sadness, silence and fear are related to a combination of stricture and laxity. Treatment should be carried out in a quiet, well-lighted and warm room, without pictures on the wall. They might stimulate the patient to experience visual hallucinations. Physical restraint may become necessary and one should guard against a patient jumping out of the window. The attendants should avoid arguing with the patient. Oil should be put on the abdomen and on the head. Venesection and cupping are indicated as well as laxatives and clysters. Food should be easily digestible and wine avoided.

The chronic diseases include mania and melancholia. Mania is an impairment of reason, without fever, occurring in young and middle

15 With availability of DRABKIN's translation an intensive study of the books of CAELIUS AURELIANUS (op. cit.) becomes possible which might clarify the psychiatric contributions of ASCLEPIADES and SORANUS.

aged men, rarely in women. It is an excessive relaxing of the mind. Many causes are given, including frequent drunkeness, sexual excess, drugs, intense studying, strong emotions of anger, grief and anxiety, suppression of menses and removal of longstanding hemorrhoids. Imminent signs are sleep disorders, unhappiness, dread and the conviction of becoming insane. The signs of the illness are impairment of reason, anger, elation or sadness and futility, dread and fear. The course is continuous or remittant, with or without forgetfulness for the psychotic experience. The patients may express delusions of being a sparrow, a cock, an earthen vessel, a God, an orator, a tragic or comic actor, a baby, or of occupying the center of the universe. SORANUS postulated that mania is chiefly physical in origin and is due to an affection of the soul.

Melancholia occurs in middle aged men and rarely in women. It is an illness which involves a state of stricture and sometimes a state of looseness and is not caused by black bile. The signs are mental anguish, dejection, animosity toward members of the household, and suspicion of a plot. The patient may weep without reason, mutter, or show joviality, longing for death, or desire to live. The physical signs are bad odors, abdominal distension, vomiting yellow and black matter and passage of discolored stool.

The treatment in all mental disorder is fundamentally the same, but in mania and melancholia the distraction of the patient and some suitable occupation is also recommended. Other physicians of this period advised intensive bleeding (to which ASCLEPIADES was opposed), flogging (TITUS 1st C. B.D.), music (ASCLEPIADES) and wine to the amount of producing drunkeness. The therapeutic value of sexual intercourse was disputed.

From his study of the course of the illness, ARETAEUS[16] (ca. 150–200 A.D.), an excellent clinician and clear writer, assumed that melancholia may be an early stage of mania. He observed also that patients who suffer from chronic melancholia the greater part of their lives became silly and behaved disgracefully. Others lacked emotional responsiveness and became fatuous, ignorant and forgetful. Mania had an intermittent course, with imperfect or complete recovery. These patients often heard noises or trumpets and pipes.

16 ARETAEUS was mentioned in the literature of the 16th and later centuries. His observation that melancholic patients have the power to predict the future was still accepted in the 16th century.

GALEN's psychiatric theories and observations are mainly presented in Book VI, but additional presentations and references are found in other volumes[17]. He states that morbid changes of mental functions do not only come from the parts which are similarly affected but also from other parts. It is easy to treat a special part which is affected and gives pain but in mental disorders there are no such indications. An impairment of the memory, for instance, is caused jointly by a damage to reason and memory and the diathesis is the same in both, but more intense in insanity where reason is lost with memory. Bilious and warm diseases cause insomnia, delirium and phrenitis. In contrast, phlegmatic and cold diseases produce torpor and drowsiness. Sluggish mental functions are caused primarily by cold and secondarily by humidity. Coma results if cold and considerable humidity are combined. Without humidity, symptoms of mania (insania) and disturbance of memory became manifest. Decreased and increased humidity and cold, and also decreased or increased dryness and warmth result in a large variety of psychopathological symptoms. Dyscrasias may attack the ventricles and sometimes the blood vessels of the whole brain. At other times, the humors which are disseminated through the brain substance and the center of the brain become intemperate.

In the search for the nature of the dyscrasias which cause psychic disturbances, one must find the dominant dyscrasia. In memory disturbance the cause is cold dyscrasia. Fever is always present in phrenitis and absent in mania and melancholia. The cause for the symptoms may be in the brain or, acting by sympathy, in another part of the body. If the cause is in the brain, all symptoms which relate to the brain will develop. If it is a sympathetic disorder the brain symptoms do not develop fully and disappear when the causes (outside the brain) cease to exist.

In discussing clinical pictures, GALEN does not offer detailed observations. He emphasized that in melancholia, phantastic imaginations occur. They are given in some detail because they were still quoted in the 16th century and later in the observations of physicians. A patient may believe that he is made of shell and as a consequence fearfully avoid people lest they might pulverize him. Another patient, seeing a cock crow while flapping his wings, will imitate the voice of the bird and flap his arms. Another fears that Atlas will become tired, drop the world, and destroy everyone. He wrote that there are a thousand similar ideas

17 The edition of KÜHN (op. cit.) and the translation of DAREMBERG (op. cit.) were used.

and many other symptoms. All melancholics are fearful and sad, find fault with life and hate men, but not all these patients wish to die. On the contrary, some melancholics are in constant fear of death, although at the same time desiring it. GALEN points out that, following HIPPO-CRATES, all the symptoms of melancholia can be grouped under sadness and fear. Sadness makes a patient hate the people he sees, and causes him to become worried and full of the fears of ignorant children and of men who tremble in deep darkness. The color of the black bile, like external darkness, darkens the seat of intelligence and produces fear. This frequently quoted example illustrates how the humors and temperament change the function of the soul. Another instance portrays the relationship between epilepsy and melancholia. GALEN also makes the interesting clinical observation that in epilepsy not only convulsions occur, but also impairment of intelligence. In his discussion of hysteria, he mentions many symptoms, including breathing difficulties and falling down with the arms and legs contracting. When the uterus returns to its normal position, the symptoms disappear. He also states that patients who abstain from sexual intercourse may become sad and lose their intelligence. For instance, one man, after the death of his wife, abstained from sexual contact and was depressed until he resumed an active sexual life. GALEN concluded that the retention of sperm has a greater damaging influence on the body than the retention of menstruation.

In another book[18] he discusses a stoic philosophy as a basis for mental health.

In the centuries after GALEN, several authors[19] wrote compilations which, however, do not offer new psychiatric contributions. They were

18   GALEN, *De cognoscendis curandisque animi morbis,* in Secunda classis materiam sanitatis. Venice 1556. (GALEN: On the passions and errors of the soul.) Transl. PAUL W. HARKINS (Cincinatti, Ohio 1963).

19   CELSUS is not mentioned because no reference was found in the textbooks and dissertations. The compilers ORIBASIUS, AETIUS and PAUL OF AEGINA were also not discussed by students. AETIUS is of psychiatric interest because he presented the teaching of ARCHIGENES, a student of AESCLIAPEDES who, under the heading of lupine disease separated rabies from lupine melancholia. AETIUS also included (Tetrabil. II, sermo II, cap. II) the first detailed description of lycanthropy by MARCELLUS SIDETA (2nd century):
'Those who are seized with the so-called lupine or canine disease, go out at night during the month of February, in everything imitating wolves or dogs and up until daybreak they are busy opening tombs. You will know people who are thus affected by these signs: they are pale with a weak expression and have dry eyes and do not weep. You will also see that they have hollow eyes and a dry tongue

infrequently quoted in the medical literature of the medieval and Renaissance periods[20]. The books of ALEXANDER OF TRALLES († 605) followed GALEN's teaching[21]. Mania is considered a more intense degree of melancholia. The author also mentions that melancholia, which is a chronic disease, may have periods of complete well-being.

RHAZES briefly discussed delirium (Karabit), melancholia and hysteria. His influence was obvershadowed by AVICENNA[22], who wrote a psychological treatise in which he postulated five faculties of the interior senses but emphasized that only three are important for medicine: imagination, reasoning and memory. The common sense (sensorium commune) deals with the present. It receives all images perceived and combines them into one mental picture. Imagination, located in the anterior part of the brain, preserves what has been received by the common sense. The cogitative faculty, in the mid-brain, deals with reason and judgment. The memory, in the posterior part of the brain, includes retention, reproduction and recognition of past experiences. He discussed systematically the signs of normal and abnormal psychological functioning. In this connection, he mentioned the influence of dominant humors on the brain: the sanguine humor causing pictures of blood and red colors, the choleric of fire and yellow, atrabilus of torture and black objects and fear of darkness, the serous humor of water and thunder. A plethora of humors is expressed in dreams of itching, burning and fetid odors.

and do not salivate at all. They are also thirsty and they have shinbones so ulcerated as to defy medical treatment, as a result of continual falls and dog bites. And these indeed are the signs. But one should know that this disease is a species of melancholy.'

As the disease comes on at night he advised to administer opium and moistening of the hand to induce sleep. AETIUS also stressed the importance of recognizing foolish behavior of children and adolescents which was separated from melancholia and delirium.

20   The Byzantine compilers who have discussed psychiatric disorders (ORIBASIUS, AETIUS, PAULUS OF AEGINA) and ALEXANDER OF TRALLES have not yet been studied satisfactorily. The best critical presentation is by FALK, op. cit.

21   ALEXANDER TRALLIANUS, Libri dudodecim graeci et latini, GUINTERIO ANDERNACO interprete, Basel 1556. In chapter 17 ALEXANDER states that melancholia was caused by an excessive amount of blood or by atrabilious or bilious blood. The last type is similar to manic excitement; chronic melancholia and its course is well described.

22   AVICENNA's general pathological concepts are discussed in the translation of OSKAR GRUNER, Treatise on the Canon of Medicine of Avicenna, London 1930, and his total work in the book of AFNAN (op. cit.). A review of his contribution to psychiatry must be based on the Canon (op. cit.).

The mental illnesses[23] comprise melancholia, mania and phrenitis. In a general psychopathological introduction, he discusses disorders of sleep and consciousness, of thinking and orientation to reality, of memory, of reason and judgment, and of imagination. Each illness is discussed under the headings of pathology, signs, and treatment. The signs of melancholia are sadness and the expectation of misfortune, or malicious behavior and agitation. The desire for solitude may be present. Hallucinations of fire or of brilliant red may occur, and noises, such as the sound of trumpets. There may also be disorders of thinking and judgment as well as fear, which may lead to violent anger. Anxiety with its physiological signs and abdominal complaints are explained by cerebral malfunctioning. His descriptions of fearful delusions correspond to those of GALEN, but with stress on robbers and demons and on dangerous animals (e.g., wolves), which surround habitations. In pure melancholia the patients wail, either fearing or seeking death. Another type of melancholia is characterized by lack of interest, untidiness and the need to be alone. In sanguine melancholia the patients laugh and have pleasant imaginations. Mania is a choleric type of melancholia, with symptoms of excitement, and dancing and attacking people. Similar symptoms occur in phrenitis (carabitus) and under demonological influences. Hysterical symptoms, included under diseases of the uterus, are mentioned in detail.

AVICENNA's treatment of psychiatric illnesses followed GALEN with some additional Arabic medications.

CONSTANTINUS AFRICANUS[24] presents, in a well-written discussion of melancholia, the teachings of RUFUS and GALEN. Of interest are his

---

23 AVICENNA in the *Canon medicinae*, Fen (book) I, Tract. III, cap. 1 discussed phrenitis, in Tract. IV, cap. 8 general psychopathology, cap. 11 intellectual impairment, cap. 12 disorders of memory and 14 of imagination, cap. 15 mania, cap. 18 melancholia and its subgroups of cutubut (an agitated form of depression) in cap. 22, iliscus (the secual unrest and excitement which later authors called melancholia heroica) in cap. 23 and lycanthropy in cap. 24. Hysteria is found in Fen I, Tract. IV, cap. 16.

24 RUDOLF CREUTZ and WALTER CREUTZ: '*Melancholia*' bei Konstantinus Africanus und seinen Quellen, Arch. Psychiat. Nervenkr. 97: 244 (1932). Translates CONSTANTINUS' psychiatric presentation and offers a critical evaluation of his contribution.

CONSTANTINUS refers to RUFUS EPHESIUS (fl. ca. 100 A.D.), whose works which were available to him now exist only in extracts in the books of AETIUS and RHAZES (translation by CH. DAREMBERG, Paris 1879). In his presentation, he emphasizes that in melancholia, fear and anxiety cause suspicion, but suspiciousness

stress on dietary mistakes, precipitating physical illnesses and toxic and psychological factors. He emphasizes that treatment should start with encouragement and relaxing music, and he outlines in detail the symptomatic treatment. His book had a strong influence in medieval medicine[25].

The power of mystical concepts, astrology, magic and demonology, became noticeable in the medical writers of the medieval period, but usually was treated with caution. ARNALD OF VILLANOVA and others[26] discussed the importance of counteracting witchcraft, but at the same time were critical of magic.

The Transitional Period of the 15th and 16th Centuries

The evolution of psychiatric thinking and practice from the later middle ages to the 16th century is related to medical progress in general and to changing philosophical, religious and cultural attitudes. Arabic-Galenic domination did not come to an abrupt end, nor was there a sudden increase of superstition and belief in witchcraft[27]. Related sexual unrest and deviations as well as religious and philosophical turmoil and the need for change were features of the middle ages. The influence of powerful mass reactions was expressed in the persecution of those who

may also lead to an increase of fear. When black bile affects the brain, it damages reason, resulting in difficulty in grasping what is familiar, and thus in suspiciousness and fear. Sadness comes from the loss of a beloved object and is accompanied by a foreboding of coming disaster. The emotions in melancholia may easily change from anger to gentleness, sadness to joy, fear to audacity. The physician cannot recognize the patient's changing behavior if he does not see him daily. As RUFUS had stated, before treatment can begin one must know how the illness started. Many phenomena cannot be understood except from daily conversation with the patient and from knowledge of the pre-illness personality. Starting the chapter on treatment, CONSTANTINUS emphasized that one should attempt to allay and remove suspicion, fear, and false impressions by gentle reasoning.

25   THORNDYKE, *op. cit.,* vol. II, 13th and 14th centuries.
26   ARNALD OF VILLANOVA in his *Breviarus liber quartus* discussed sexual excitement, the treatment of melancholia and remedies against demons and witchcraft. BERNARDUS DE GORDON (ca. 1318) in the *Lilium medicinae* followed, but not blindly, GALEN and the Arabic writers. GUAINERIO *(op. cit.)* shows more independence. Translations of passages from his book are found in succeeding footnotes.
27   At some universities AVICENNA's influence persisted into the 18th century and belief in demonology was strong among leading chemiatrists. SCHIPPERGES *(op. cit.)* discusses the followers of Arabic medicine in the medieval period, the 15th century and later, and the anti-Arabic movement of the 16th century.

proposed, or demanded, change and offered solutions for the misery in which people lived.

Spanish mysticism, expounded by RAYMON LULL (1235–1315) and his contemporary, ARNALDUS OF VILLANOVA, exerted a wide influence in medicine, and astrology was deemed important for prognosis and treatment. Both mysticism and astrology became strengthened by the Neoplatonism of the 15th century.

The changing role of psychiatry is well documented by GUAINERIO († 1440)[28] who, like other contemporary teachers, reconsidered AVICENNA's grouping of nine types of melancholia, resulting in a regrouping of symptoms and a recognition of separate clinical pictures. This change permitted at the beginning of the 16th century descriptions of the illnesses of individual patients in the published observations of physicians. Another step of importance was that each illness was discussed under the heading of definition, which included a review of literature, causes, demonstrable signs, their prognostic significance and treatment.

Discussing delirium, GUAINERIO stressed the importance of a complete physical study because the delirium, caused by inflammation of the brain or the meninges, may occur as a phase in other diseases (pleurisy, pneumonia) or be related to illnesses of the heart, liver, stomach, kidneys, or uterus. He emphasized that a predelirious period, caused by 'the putrid fumes from the resolution of warm humors', can be recognized which may or may not lead to a full delirium[29]. The outcome depends on the constitution of the patient, the nature of the illness to which the delirium is related, and on the treatment. He also noted that a delirium may change into melancholia, mania, and dangerous excitements.

Although he stated, like other authors of the 15th century, that mania and melancholia were separate illnesses his attitude was somewhat ambiguous. When he discussed the symptoms of melancholia he stressed the need to recognize early changes in the patient's behavior from the observations of members of the household[30]. Under the broad

---

28   GUAINERIO frequently gives credit to GALEN, ALEXANDER OF TRALLES, and CONSTANTINUS AFRICANUS as well as RHAZES and AVICENNA. The philosophers who influenced him were PLATO, ARISTOTLE and AVERROËS.

29   The term 'paraphrenitis' includes predelirium.

30   He accepts the three stages of melancholia of RHAZES. The first grade is recognized by fearfulness, sadness, love for solitude and quickness to anger without sufficient cause; the second by the patient's talk of his groundless fears and that

heading of melancholia, mania is presented as a separate entity. The extrinsic causes are the same as in melancholia, but the intrinsic causes are in the brain – 'bad quality alone or a bad quality with matter'. The symptoms are different, depending on the causes[31].

When a mixture of the humors is involved[32] GUAINERIO described a mixed affective picture which is close to the description of CONSTANTINUS and in contrast to ARETAEUS, who is credited in modern literature with having been the first author to have mentioned the manic-depressive illness.

The presentation of mania and melancholia is well organized and

something would be done to him. The third grade is reached when he 'accomplishes in deeds what he had perceived in his mind'. GUAINERIO advises:
'Through those stages you will recognize someone who has become melancholic. Such things are easily learned from those who live in the same house and are familiar with him, because when natures that are understood at the time of good health seem to change from their earlier state, you will know that they have fallen into this suffering.'
He continues this discussion by giving the example:
'If we know that someone is naturally vain, eloquent or irritable, and this vanity, eloquence or temper have been violently altered, we say in the case of such a man that he is mentally ill, and contrariwise of a timid man turned irritable and bold.' (Tract 15, III.).
In this statement GUAINERIO is clearly influenced by CONSTANTINUS.
31 'If it is only a bad quality, the patient himself will fear everything indifferently because he will be terrified especially by dead people, black and shadowy things, and talk of such things.' ... 'Where matter is responsible the patient feels heaviness. Headache, scotoma, vertigo, insomnia and other ills of the head have preceded. He often fixes his gaze on one spot, and becomes angry if anyone tries to remove him from it. He loves solitude more than others. He perseveres in intense thought. This will be an especially strong indication if you observe that all his other members are in good health.
'But if the faulty humor is bloodly melancholy, the acts of the patient will be marked by laughter and joy and he will like spacious, bright and happy places like meadows and gardens and he will desire to enjoy such things along with friends. He takes pleasure in musical melodies, and so, in sum, this melancholy is marked by very little sadness in comparison with the others.' (Tract. 15, III.)
32 'Sometimes bile is burned up along with the blood. This kind now fears, now laughs, now quarrels, and briefly the acts of the burned-up blood and the burned-up bile, as ALEXANDER [OF TRALLES] says, are mixed with each other. And thus it happens if burned-up blood is mixed with melancholia, because the patients now laugh, now weep, now rejoice, now fear, and so goes the mixture in the rest of their acts.' (Tract. 15, III.)

the clinical observations are stressed in a way which is representative of the 16th century[33].

When GUAINERIO cautioned against being guided in treatment by the astrological rules, he was more critical than his contemporaries[34]. He takes a similar attitude to the teaching that melancholics could foretell the future or illiterates become literate in a state of melancholia[35].

Sexual unrest of the 14th and succeeding centuries was only briefly mentioned in medical books. The well-known behavior of patients, especially women, in dancing mania illustrates some of the psychopathology of sexual excitements. Although the widespread epidemics of dancing manias of the 13th and 14th centuries had come to an end, sporadic

33   Looking retrospectively at GUIANERIO's groupings we can recognize mania, depression, mixed manic-depressive states, schizophrenia and mild mood reactions which were included in KRAEPELIN's classification at the end of the 19th century. It is interesting to note GUAINERIO's omission of lycanthropy, which was mentioned by the authors of the previous centuries as well as those of the Renaissance, when under the Neoplatonic influence metempsychosis was re-accepted. He calls a mania 'lupine' if the patient has the ferocity of a wolf; struggling, striking, biting.
'The common people, and especially ignorant monks, say that such a one has a wolf-devil in him.' (Tract. 15, III.)
34   'You need not take observations of the light of the moon, nor the aspects of the other planets, provided everything else is amenable to a phlebotomy. Do not let the same thing happen to you that happened to a friend of mine during such days: he postponed performing a phlebotomy on a strong delirious person until the moon had gone through its phase. On account of this the delirium was strengthened in the interim and the symptoms increased, for the good man while singing a song passed into eternal life.' (Tract. 3, VI.)
35   These claims of ALEXANDER [OF TRALLES] and RHAZES are treated by GUAINERIO from the point of view of scholastic philosophy. He mentions briefly that he had seen a farmer who, he was told, had never learned to read or write. This farmer 'composed songs during the combustion of the moon'. In a lengthy discussion, after a further review of medical literature, he presents five suppositions to state and prove that the soul's dominant star can pour its influence into the soul when the soul is free of the impending mediation of the sense. This freedom is achieved in the ecstasy of melancholia. Hence melancholia is an occasion of extraordinary acquisition of knowledge. The author then proposes two arguments against this conclusion, which he afterwards refutes (HEFFERNAN). He states that he offers this theoretical discussion as defense against charges [from philosophers] that a physician does not understand the causes that befall men. His final sentence disposes of the value of such a discussion:
'And thus far on the problem, the causes of which, when assigned bring serious difficulties after them. I relinquish them to theoreticians, and pass on to the glories of practice of medicine.' (Tract. 15, IV.)

cases were seen in the 16th century. PARACELSUS described salacitas as a frequent illness of his period. GUAINERIO considered the topic[36] of sexual excitements important enough to give considerable space to a discussion of it.

During the 14th and 15th centuries economic instability, with severe unemployment and poverty, led to periods of anxiety. Superstitious hopes gave rise to religious sects, and fear turned people against the Jews, whom they attacked[37]. The repeated occurrence of dreaded epidemics, accompanied by great fear of their unknown cause and the means of

36   The Latin term *amatorius* or *cupidinerius* was substituted by AVICENNA by *hilliscus*. ARNALD OF VILLANOVA in his tractatus de heroyeo (Opera ... *superrime revisa*, Lyons 1520) used the term 'hereos'. GUAINERIO defines hereos as 'a continual imagination of something inordinately loved'.
'For our purposes *hereos* can be thus defined: *hereos* is the continual thought of the beloved or the lover, through which, under the command of the erring estimative power, an immoderate desire to obtain the object of affection is born.' ...
'The state of mind of those in *hereos* seems to be insanity since they neglect everything else and think continually of the one they love because they have an immoderate desire of obtaining the beloved.' ... 'This illness occurs in fleshy men whose warm testicles abound greatly in semen and who lead a life of idleness and pleasure. Anger, sadness and other psychological symptoms have to be dealt with. The same may occur in women. Therefore when the carnal woman leads a life of idleness and pleasure, if an attractive man meets her and she considers that he will readily comply with her wishes, she is easily caught by her sexual desires.'
[The victim of hereos] 'remains in continual deep thought, eating and drinking little and staying awake too much. He longs to be alone and when anyone distracts him from his thoughts he is angry. He sometimes weeps, and sometimes is angry and laughs. And if you announce something sad about his beloved he is saddened. If it is something pleasant, he is delighted. Unless you give help to the poor man, he will day by day waste away and be consumed, and finally vainly calling out in tears to his beloved, he will commend his unhappy soul to the guardianship of his God.' (Tract. 15, XIII.)
The most effective cure is for the patient to 'possess his beloved'. Helpful, also, are phlebotomy and purgatives and various means of distracting the patient. He closes the therapeutic discussion with a detailed description of how monks try to abolish sexual desires by chastisement, and leaves it to the reader as to whether he prefers this or the medical procedure.
37   Among the sects which attracted a large following and added greatly to social instability were the flagellantes which still existed in the 15th century when in Germany they were burnt as heretics. The 'free spirit movement' which permitted sexual freedom lasted from the 12th into the 15th century. The people's crusade of HANS BÖHM started in 1476 and later Anabaptism became widespread in Southern Germany and Switzerland. The members had ecstatic experiences and women threw themselves on the ground in hysterical-like convulsions.

their dissemination, terrorized mankind. Their outbreaks led to panic, fanatic religious revival, to an excess of pleasure-seeking and uncontrolled sexual activities.

In these periods superstitious beliefs in demonology and witchcraft increased. Although magic and, to some extent, demonology had been accepted in Arabic medicine, lycanthropy, incubus and other superstitions were explained on a psychopathological basis. The Arabic use of amulets and incantations was less favored by physicians of the 15th century, but remained a popular therapeutic tool.

The fear of demonological influences and of witches became increasingly notable in the 14th and 15th centuries[38]. Prosecutors supported accusations taken from demonological influences found in the Old Testament and in the lives of saints. The physicians seem to have stood aside and the medical books do not deal with the rapidly increasing psychological epidemic[39]. The change from a quiet acceptance of demonology to a frank and critical rejection came gradually.

In the middle ages Jews and members of certain sects were accused of killing new-born babies. In Bern several men and women were found guilty in 1430 and burnt. Some years later similar accusations were made in Strasbourg.

38   The burning of witches occurred in France (Poitou 1453, Artois 1459), and a few years later in Germany (Mainz, Trier, Salzburg). Many factors contributed to the spreading of these beliefs, less marked in Italy than in the Northern countries where many superstitions persisted among the inhabitants of isolated and mountainous regions.

39   The difficulties with which the critical physician was confronted becomes obvious in the 16th century when, e.g., FERNEL in his earlier years accepted the influence of demonological forces. One reason for the hesitancy on the part of physicians to reject demonology aggressively may have been the changing picture of psychopathology which was related to the marked individual suggestibility of the accused and on-lookers, to mass suggestibility, and religious attitudes. Toxic factors caused by the use of herbs may have played a confusing role. In the 16th century, drugs from the Mediterranian countries prescribed in Arabic medicine were found in plants and the fruits of bushes in Germany and France. Among them were some which have a strong toxic effect on the central nervous system, especially atropa belladonna (solanum niger), datura stramonium (thorn apple), hyoscyamus niger (black henbane), aconitum napellas (buttercup), cannabis sativa (hemp) and opium. The 'witches' brew' may have contained all or some of these herbs and fruits, in varying strengths, affecting participants through consumption by mouth or the inhalation of fumes. The expected effect would have been increased by verbal suggestions and mystical rituals. In a practicing 'witch' and victim, the excitement of exposing oneself to a dreadful danger, to committing a great sin, to being caught or to succeed without being caught, would have been especially strong in the young, the emotionally unstable, the fanatics. Anybody ac-

Treatment, through the 17th century remained dominated by Arabic and Galenic medicine, and is well described by GATINARIA († 1496). The essential points which a physician must always keep in mind were: (1) administration of the regimen of the six non-naturals (air, food and drink, rest and exercise, sleep and waking, excretion and retention, mental affections), (2) regulation and correction of digestion, (3) evacuation to achieve the drawing off of melancholic humors, (4) diversion of the disturbing humors from the brain and heart, (5) resolution of the residue of the black humors, and (6) strengthening of the brain and heart[40].

cused of witchcraft must have been in a state of intense fear in which he might become highly suggestible to skillful questioning and insinuations by the frightful inquisition, all this aggravated by the dreaded torture and practically unavoidable death. Increased suggestibility, in the setting of religious doubts and general insecurity, would be present in a population which suffered from undernourishment, acute and chronic infectious diseases, and from toxic factors in the environment, e.g., housing, or in industrial activities. The toxic effect might have directly affected the brain or resulted in hysterical reactions and mass psychopathology, or affect existing psychotic pictures of depressions, schizophrenic and paranoid fanatics.

In the 16th century, real and superstitious dangers became intensified by the printing of broadleafs, containing a picture with a brief statement under it, describing some dreadful event with superstitious exaggeration, e.g., violent storms, the appearance of a comet, murder, hangings, and evil deeds by the devil and witches (FEHR, *op. cit.*).

40   GATINARIA (*op. cit*) outlines the treatment:

1. Regimen of the six non-naturals (air, food and drink, rest and exercise, sleep and waking, excretion and retention, mental affections) – it was considered especially important to have moisture and also warmth. The air should be kept moist with vases full of water, and kept warm by the addition of marsh mallows. The flowers should give a pleasant odor. Food should omit too much salt. Chicken broth is highly recommended. Much rest is necessary; (others recommend well-planned physical activity). Sleep, which is usually disturbed or decreased, can be induced by a warm bath, rubbing oil on the temples, a light massage with syrup of poppies or violets in lettuce water. Opium may be needed for marked insomnia but must be given carefully, and omitted in patients who do not have good strength. Even in light cases of melancholia, attention must be paid to healthy digestion, good excretion and avoidance of disturbing emotions.

2. Regulation and correction of digestion were accomplished by the use of syrups of thyme, epithyme, fruits and bugloss water (used in cordials).

3. Evacuation to achieve the drawing off melancholic humors by bleeding, diaphoretics, purgation, diuretics. Light cathartics, e.g., rhubarb, were recommended at the beginning of the illness. Strong purgatives were considered indicated for marked depression and included senna and black hellebore.

4. Diversion of the disturbing humors from the brain and heart were achieved by moderate bleeding from the legs, using preferably the left vena basilica as well as

The increasing questioning of Arabic authorities in the 15th century prepared the way for modern medicine by increasing attention on careful clinical observations and their critical analysis. In the field of normal human behavior one must mention JUAN LUIS VIVES (1492–1540), who supported his psychological discussions with graphic observations[41], stressing the role of emotions on memory and intellectual functions. In the leading medical books of this era, a valuable listing of symptoms and reference to the course of the illness are found, but are usually too concise to permit an appraisal of their significance from the point of view of current psychiatry. The earliest book of a collection of observations on psychiatric disorders from many authors, as well as his own practice, was published by FORESTUS, *op. cit.*[42].

cupping glasses. If the blood seemed black it should be withdrawn but not if it was clear and thin. Scarification was also used. Clysters were recommended. Diversion was also accomplished by binding the arms and legs, and massaging the hips. 5. Resolution of the residue of the black humors is accomplished by external application to achieve moistening.

Phlebotomy deserves some discussion. Blood should be withdrawn to achieve evacuation, to help diversion, to preserve good health or for diagnostic purpose. Copious bleeding was indicated in excitements of various types; moderate bleeding for diversion, e. g., in delirium and in marked pain. In Arabic medicine bleeding and venesection were as far removed from the diseased part as possible. PIERRE BRISSOT (1478–1522) attacked this teaching and, due to his influence, the advice of HIPPOCRATES was followed to perform the venesection close to the lesion. (In the dissertations either method was recommended.) The indications for copious bleeding in psychiatric conditions were not affected by the doctrine involved.

41 In *De anima et vita* (1538) VIVES in general follows ARISTOTLE and GALEN. Psychiatrically, his discussion of memory and the role of emotions on retention and recall is especially interesting. He describes in some detail the process how one idea recalls another. In his lengthy discussion of emotions he stresses the physiological aspect as well as offering an accurate description of specific emotions. The variety of emotions are grouped under the drives to pursue good and avoid evil. His *De subventione pauperum* (1525) contains in book II, chapter 3, a strong plea for the humane treatment of psychotic patients in hospitals and at home. His direct influence on psychiatric thinking cannot be evaluated. As far as I know, he is not referred to in the texts of medical writers. References: RAYMOND D. CLEMENTS, *The role of J. L. Vives in the development of modern medical science.* Diss. U. Chicago 1964, and *Physiological-psychological thought in Juan Luis Vives,* J. Hist. Behav. Sci., vol. 3, 1967. GERHARD HOPPE, *Die Psychologie des Juan Luis Vives.* Diss. Erlangen 1901.

42 Consultations (Consultationes and Epistolae) which were published are of limited value because the clinical data are meager. Sometimes their discussion is interesting because it illustrates the author's theoretical point of view and the treatment suggested which, however, usually followed GALEN and Arabic teaching.

In the succeeding chapters of this book, the value of clinical observation to which dissertations have made a valuable contribution, becomes manifest.

Chapter III
Melancholia

The term 'melancholia' includes a large group of psychiatric illnesses which can be divided into depressive and schizophrenic illnesses. The catatonic illnesses were not included in melancholia but were treated as a separate entity.

1. Depressions

The definition of melancholia, in the depressive sense, is based on GALEN and has been largely modified by Arabic authors. Later, the dissertations refer to the authorities of PLATTER, SENNERT, DU LAURENS, RIVIÈRE, WILLIS and BOERHAAVE.

GALEN's teaching is well represented by the early dissertations of Basel. THONER (Basel 1590) states: 'By the term melancholic disorder we denote that disease in which the imagination is depraved with fear and sadness.' Something happens to the brain 'by means of which a shadowy phantasm arises' which corrupts the seat of imagination and sometimes of reason. A melancholic delirium (i.e., delusions) is 'the depravity of the principal function along with fear and sadness'. The cause of the shadowy phanthasm can bei either external ('when a man is saddened and made fearful without manifest cause') or internal. If this is the case melancholia is 'a sympathetic reaction from the whole' or originates in the hypochondrium which includes the 'stomach, the spleen, the mesenteries, the uterus, but it is always necessary that the upper mouth of the stomach be affected in the disease since there is a remarkable sympathetic reaction between the mouth of the stomach and the brain'. Oncoming melancholy can be foretold from 'wakefulness, disturbed and restless sleep with sad images, sluggishness of the whole body, fatigue in talking, along with overclouded eyes'. PESTALOZZI (Basel 1615) formulated the same theory in a modified form explaining the three kinds of melancholia according to GALEN in the following statements:

'The first [kind of melancholia] comes from melancholic, gross and filthy blood congested in the brain itself' – 'the second is stirred up when all the veins of the body are flooded with melancholic blood' – 'the third kind of melancholy, called hypochondriacal, depends on a cold imbalance of the intestines and the stomach.'

The external causes are unhealthy air, diet, exercise, sleep and the retention of evacuations, especially hemorrhoidal and menstrual blood. The internal causes

'include a cold and dry imbalance of the brain from a melancholic humor and its vapors, contained in the head or in the whole body and generated there or transmitted from elsewhere. Since they are black and turbulent, they also render the animal spirits foul and turbulent, whence, GALEN writes that it happens that, just as boys are terrified by external darkness, so on account of the shadowy constitution of the brain, the principal faculty of the mind is disturbed in its operation'. 'At other times melancholy is also a disease of the spleen when it attracts a large mass of this kind of raw blood and does not purge it out. This we see in suppressed menstrual flow and suppressed hemorrhoids and in the excrement of the blood which is regurgitated both into the whole body and up to the very seat of the mind.'

These statements illustrate how little these theories of GALEN were affected by the teachings of PLATTER whose students wrote the above dissertations. His contribution was in making the students aware of the clinical picture.

In the dissertation of UNVERZAGT (Helmstadt 1614) GALEN's theory is supported: primary melancholia has

'as its subject the brain only. The disorder in this case would arise from actual imbalance in the brain itself, or from causes which generate melancholic matters in the brain, e.g., worry, fear, frightening sights, violent imagination and wakefulness'.

Secondary melancholy

'arises out of imbalance or disorder in some part other than the brain but which is concerned with the production of blood, for example, the liver'. 'A third species has as its seat the hypochondrium, whence a dark and smoky vapor is transmitted to the brain.'

UNVERZAGT discusses ARGENTERIUS[1] critically. He stresses that in dreams, as well as in melancholia, the same phanthasms, coming from the same disposition of spirits, cause bizarre imaginations. In Helmstadt,

1 ARGENTERIUS, JOHANNES, *De somno et vigilia,* Florence 1556.

where LIDDELL had taught from 1596–1607, the critical study of literature seems to have been more encouraged than in the far more outstanding Department of Medicine in Basel. This impression may be erroneous and should be clarified by a study of this aspect of medical education. LIDDELL's own dissertation *De melancholia* (Helmstadt 1596) which is classed with schizophrenic illnesses, as well as dissertations which were written under him, illustrate the use of literature in the 16th and early 17th centuries.

SENNERT, still quoted in the 18th century, postulated that the cause of idiopathic melancholia is in the brain itself whereas in sympathetic melancholia (identical with symptomatic melancholia) the cause is in some other part of the body. The prognosis was considered better for symptomatic than idiopathic melancholia (SCHEFFER, Helmstadt 1652).

The influence of WILLIS brought about a change in theories and this is well illustrated in the dissertation of VATER (Wittenberg 1680) which will be discussed below. BOERHAAVE's teaching is recognizable in Oos-TERDYCK-SCHACH's dissertation (Leyden 1693). He criticized GALEN's triple classification of melancholia and proposed instead the distinction of melancholia with and without matter, i.e. faulty humor, the first type he called hysterical, or nervous, melancholia which is inherent in the brain. Melancholia, caused by a humoral disorder, may be universal (atrabilious) or in a particular part of the body (hypochondriacal melancholia).

The clinical division into three types of melancholia, originated with GALEN and persisted in various forms. Usually, however, the clinical division only described depression characterized by sadness, feelings of anxiety and fearful preoccupations (including delusions) and hypochondriacal anxiety. Following DU LAURENS[2], others distinguished three types by stressing the intensity of the depression. Thus, SCHEFFER (Helmstadt 1652) describes type 1 as characterized by being sad, morose and adverse to social contact. Type 2 has, in addition to these symptoms, horrible imaginings, fear of dangers and wandering about trying to avoid them. In type 3 one finds delusional talk and actions caused by delusions. The melancholia may develop into furor and degenerate into mania (see chapter V). This development is simlar to the concept of the course of melancholia as accepted at the end of the 18th century. Another attempt at classification tries to relate the psychopathological symp-

2   DU LAURENS, *op. cit.*

toms to specific organs. FUCHS (Jena 1671) and NEUSE (Jena 1685) emphasize that the brain as a whole is affected by melancholy (MERCURIALIS[3] taught that the front part of the brain, concerned with reason, was affected, ARNALDUS VILLANOVA[4] that it was the middle part where imagination resides). The affected spirits and blood carry the emotional impression which causes an expansion or tightening of the heart. This fact is demonstrated by the symptoms of anxiety. This reasoning of the authors is the same as VAN HELMONT's[5] who, observing frequent spitting of melancholics, concluded that the stomach was involved. The cause of melancholy is the unnatural concentration of blood and spirits. The primary subject of melancholy is the brain, the secondary the whole body, and in particular, the heart. The melancholic humors are generated and contained in the mesenteric veins, the spleen and liver, the genitals, the hypochondrium, the heart and the substance of the brain.

Students continued to look critically at these questions, quoting and questioning established authorities, under the influence of the progress of medicine as expressed by new observations and theories. In 1728, BÖNNEKEN (Erfurt) covered the topic in detail. In his definition he included the significance of emotions and the course of the illness. Delusions may be present continuously or at intervals. He pointed out that the illness may have physical, or moral, causes, or both simultaneously. The results may be a sad, or cheerful, melancholia. Violent emotional experiences may precipitate the illness, as well as religious fears and guilt. The relationship of emotions and physical symptoms is reviewed in detail. Thus, this dissertation offers a good orientation to the psychiatric thinking of the first quarter of the 18th century and offers much information about literature.

In the field of depression the dissertations offer few clinical observations, quoting usually those of PLATTER, DU LAURENS, DIEMERBROECK[6]. Frequently the authors are not even mentioned because their descriptions, by their frequent quoting, have become undisputed facts which do not need to be evaluated critically. It reminds one of the scholastic attitude to data offered by GALEN and Arabic authors. The lack of case contributions is most regretable because only a careful description of the emotional symptoms permits a reader to decide whether delusions and

---

3   MERCURIALIS, op. cit. and De arte gymnastica, Venice 1573.
4   ARNALDUS OF VILLANOVA, op. cit.
5   HELMONT, JOANNE BAPTISTA VAN, Ortus medicinae, Amsterdam 1652.
6   DIEMERBROECK, op. cit.

hallucinations are depressive, or schizophrenic, in nature. It is likely that most of the delusions, which were described in the observations of the above-mentioned authors, occurred in a depressive illness. The diagnostic decision is difficult because the course of an illness is frequently not mentioned. The importance of the development and final outcome was not fully appreciated until the end of the 17th century.

The delusions repeatedly quoted which are most likely depressive in nature are those mentioned by DU LAURENS (1598)[7]: Some relate to the body such as being made of glass, of having a snake in the stomach, of going to be changed into a bird. Another type is related to the mode of living, e.g., being wealthy or a king, or having lost all wealth.

There is little about the clinical picture of depressions to be added by dissertations to PLATTER's description in the chapter on melancholia in his textbook.

SCHEFFER (Helmstadt 1652) stresses the important point that a depressed patient may show distorted judgment when dealing with his delusions but he may judge correctly otherwise. He quotes FORESTUS (book X, observation 15):

'A learned merchant was troubled with a false imagination that he had lost all his property (although he was very rich) and that he was damned and could feel the pains of Hell, although in every other respect he reasoned correctly, read books and discussed their content with FORRESTUS.'

SCHEFFER remarks later that the 'melancholics are timid and the timid are suspicious. They easily imagine things, especially if the mind is under a strain'. The victims of a depressive illness are morose and pensive, often suspicious and have delusions, e.g., of being a chicken, an earthenware vessel.

The signs of depression are well presented by RHENANUS (Marburg 1615) who follows the teachings of GALEN and PLATTER. He stresses that the illness is characterized by sadness and fear with disturbed imagination and intact reasoning and memory. Dependent on the extent of the damage to the imagination, reasoning may be affected. The affect of emotions on reasoning is acknowledged but not stressed. The outstanding emotions are sorrow and fear, timidity and despair (despite wealth, honors, and fortune). The patients become taciturn, their heads bowed to the ground, desiring to be alone, weary of their daily life. They show a lack of desire to do things. They sleep poorly, and are restless and

7   DU LAURENS, op. cit.

fearful when awake. This description fits a depressed patient but also some schizophrenics.

The best review of early literature is offered by DU MONT (Helmstadt 1659) who follows GALEN and the Arabic writers, turns to ZACUTUS LUSITANUS[8] and PLATTER and includes the observations of HEER, FOREST and SOLENANDER[9]. The author includes elation, schizophrenic, as well as depressive illnesses, but keeps them well separated. The development of a broader interest in these illnesses in the second part of the 17th century can be seen in the dissertation of HAENDTSCHKY (Wittenberg 1702), who offers additional references with regard to delusions, behavior and thinking.

As has been mentioned previously, delusions are discussed frequently although not sufficiently described. Hallucinations are visual in nature; very rarely are they auditory. Depressed patients are frightened by the appearance of ghosts and dead people, and less frequently by demons. The case of DIEMERBROECK[10] (chap. III, p. 4) is quoted – a 48-year-old man in a deep depression has delusions of being possessed and experiences visual hallucinations. Paranoid delusions in depressions attracted early attention. FISCHER (Helmstadt 1607) summarizes them well. He included lycanthropy in depression, accepting the teachings of WIERUS and CAMERARIUS. It is interesting to note that the interest in lycanthropy (by Arabic writers called cutubuth) waned after the 16th century. There are no dissertations on this topic but references to it are found in discussions of demonology (see chap. IX). Another aspect of depression, the intense agitation and fear, which was described as a definite illness and frequently referred to by the Arabic writers under the term 'cutubuth' or 'melancholia errabunda', attracted passing attention in the 17th century.

The authors, in textbooks and dissertations, separate anxiety from fear. Anxiety already was noticed among the early symptoms of depression. This observation confirmed the opinion that the heart as well as the brain was involved. Fear, with well-defined objects causing the reaction, was found in more intense or advanced stages of depression. These topics are discussed at various lengths in many dissertations.

The different ages in which depressions occur were considered, but no definite differentiations were offered. Occasionally the involutional

8   ZACUTUS LUSITANUS, *op. cit.*
9   SOLENANDER, *op. cit.*, sect. V, cons. XVII.
10   DIEMERBROECK, *op. cit.*, Disputationes practicae case III and IV.

phase was mentioned but not discussed at length. More interesting was the relationship of menstruation to depression, because amenorrhea signified a serious disturbance in the evacuation of a melancholie humor. The dissertation of CRELLIUS (Leipzig 1732) summarizes well the attitude of previous authors.

SCHULTZ (Frankfurt a. O. 1705) studied post-partum reactions and reviewed literature with special attention to the sparse clinical observations. He limited this type of melancholia, which was called melancholia *ex utero* or also hysterica, to post-partum psychoses without fever and excitement, thus excluding toxic psychoses caused by infection. He presented his observation of a depressive post-partum psychosis. The depression occurred in a 20-year-old woman on the 6th day after delivery. Her depression was characterized by insomnia, marked anxiety and desperate thoughts about which she talked a great deal. The physician described at length the physical treatment. BERGER (Göttingen 1745) discussed mania and melancholia in the puerperium.

As I have mentioned previously, little attention is given to prognosis and course of the illness. SCHEFFER (Helmstadt 1652) stresses that hereditary, or constitutional, melancholy is cured with difficulty whereas an acute case is easily cured. Melancholy, which is contracted from a disorder of the spleen and uterus, is more easily cured than that which comes from disorders of the heart (i.e., with marked anxiety). He gives a better prognosis if the imagination alone is injured: it is more serious if the reason is also affected (i.e., a pure depression has a better prognosis than if schizophrenic symptoms are present). He states that mania arises from melancholia when wet and dry conditions form a combination.

The relationship of depressions to excitements has been noted in the observations of medical writers, e.g. FABRICIUS HILDANUS[11] and SCHENCK[12] and confirmed in a thesis by GORION (Paris 1600). In reading such references one has to keep in mind that melancholia included schizophrenia and depression, and manic excitements, which might be schizophrenic or manic. The statement by VATER (Wittenberg 1680) that 'mania and melancholia often change into one another' might refer to schizophrenia during a phase of excitement. However, as VATER discussed a psychosis characterized by sadness (delirium triste), one might be justified in thinking of a manic-depressive illness. He wrote:

11 FABRICIUS HILDANUS, *op. cit.,* centuria IV, obs. IX.
12 SCHENCK, *op. cit.,* lib. I, de melancholia, obs. III.

'Melancholia often passes into mania and vice versa. The melancholics themselves now laugh, now are saddened, now express numberless other absurd gestures and forms of behavior.'

VATER, who later became an outstanding teacher and supervised a
large number of valuable dissertations, made the critical remark:

'It is vain to look to humors, or spirits, for an explanation of this [change
into one another].'

STANGIUS (Halle 1700) referred to the relationship of melancholia
and mania without further elucidation, nor did BOERHAAVE with his
statement that if mania results from melancholia, reaches such 'a height
as to agitate the juices of the brain' (Aphorism 1118).

The treatment closely follows the outlines given in the textbooks.
An interesting presentation is offered by BACMEISTER and PAULI (Rostock 1593). BACMEISTER's propositions defend GALEN's theory of melancholia, also, including the teachings of AVICENNA and AVERRHOES. This
presentation was followed by PAULI's propositions on treatment. He discusses all the aspects in detail, and in a special section the treatment of
hypochondriacal melancholia. This combined presentation offers an interesting glimpse of the teaching in the German medical schools of the
16th century.

The dissertation of FLACHT (Basel 1620) offers a systematic discussion of PLATTER's treatment recommending the herbs and drugs to be
used for alterantia (alternatives to affect the melancholic humors), for
evacuation, for corroborantia (strengthening the brain) and errhina (to
excite sneezing and to increase nasal mucous). For external application
fomentation (partial bathing), embroche (irrigation of the head), lini-
ments and bath are indicated. In marked symptoms, and especially in
hypochondriacal melancholy, purgation induced vomiting and surgical
procedures (venesection, and the other previously mentioned procedures) are needed.

A more sophisticated presentation of treatment, although demonstrating little fundamental progress, is offered by FUCHS (Jena 1671).
His dissertation is well written, and includes much reference material
and practical advice.

A critical review of therapy is offered by CAPAULIS (Leyden 1665),
with regard to the effect of hemorrhoidal discharge. He admits that this
loss of blood seems to be helpful in melancholia:

'I confess that it is difficult to explain the small hemorrhoidal flux–why it is comforting to the sick. I was never present at such a case to examine all the circumstances of the blood loss. This is the kind of thing which practitioners pass by ... Looking at both sides, therefore, I am of the opinion that this flux provides some relief to the sick person.'

Reviewing the literature on melancholia the following points become obvious: The pathognomic symptoms are sadness and fear. The common sensorium is affected. There may be many or few symptoms enumerated, but not well described. Hallucinations are usually described as phanthasm. Etiologically, the distinctions are made between idiopathic and symptomatic melancholia and between contracted and hereditary. The course may be continuous with remissions and exacerbations, or just intermittent (periodic). In other cases happiness may be replaced by sadness. The findings on the involvement of the spleen and the concept of black bile were questioned with the increasing knowledge of pathological anatomy.

2. The Hypochondriacal Depression

A summary of PLATTER offers the basic clinical teaching at the beginning of the 17th century[13]. Hypochondriacal melancholia, which has its origin in the spleen and mesenteric veins, gives pain and discomfort to the patient. His clinical description might well fit the picture of hypochondriasis as described 80 years later by HIGHMORE:

'The symptoms described are very often intermittent, often recurring the same day. Those who suffer from it ... know that they are really sick. (Herein they suffer from others who, unless some further symptom has acceded, complain only of headaches or heaviness of the head.) Although they hardly ever lie down, and can nonetheless perform their other duties, still they complain of a continual pain especially on their left side (which they call heart pain), of sweating, of pulse, of rumbling in the bowels, belching, vomiting, expectorations, headache, vertigo, ringing in their ears, throbbing arteries, and other innumerable disorders which they feel and which they imagine. They importune their doctors, beg for cures, try various remedies, and, unless they are soon relieved, they change their doctors and their drugs.'

In his *Observationes* he describes in detail the treatment. He mentions that educated people

13   F. PLATTER, *op. cit.,* p. 86.

'Especially those who are engaged in the study of medicine, and from investigating the causes of diseases, think that any change in the body, even the most trivial, is a sign of something wrong and proceeds from some disease'.

Patients often complain

'That they have lost all their natural heat ... and that their brain, stomach, lungs, liver, kidneys, and in women, the uterus, has been weakened and disordered and has become full of excrement, when, in truth, there is no trouble at all but merely a melancholy imagination'.

He later states that some patients, who complain about an abdominal disorder, suffer from some real hypochondriac disorders but, in addition, imagine many other things. PLATTER's sound medical attitude had no doubt a far-reaching influence.

The earliest dissertation on hypochondriacal melancholia, also called melancholia flatuosa, was presented by RENTZIUS (Tübingen 1594). The hypochondriacal depression also received considerable attention in dissertations on melancholia, e.g., by BORNEMANN (Basel 1594). An attempt to offer a better description was made by BRUXIUS (Basel 1604) and BATTUS (Basel 1605). BRUXIUS stressed the psychopathological picture, giving a good description of the behavior of the worried and anxious patient, filled by terrors, often unable to express himself freely. His memory and imagination may be affected. His main preoccupations are the abdominal symptoms and palpitations. The author warned against not noticing an underlying organic abdominal disease. BATTUS emphasized this possibility in the presence of the symptoms of depression and undue anxiety about health, vomiting, eructation and flatulence. Like other authors he followed the previously outlined treatment. COLERUS (Basel 1608) stressed the importance of the combination of physical illnesses and depression. He reviewed scorbut, the ill-defined and common nutritional disorders of the period. This dissertation is further discussed in the chapter on hypochondriasis. Interest in the abdominal illnesses and depression continued at the Basel faculty. The dissertation of MELANCHTHON (Basel 1629) contributed little that was new while CRUSIUS (Basel 1645) discussed in greater detail the psychopathological findings. He singled out the disturbances of imagination and reasoning, and the occurrence of delusions. The treatment was reviewed at length, but was essentially the same as that previously outlined.

RIVIÈRE (1640)[14] states that 'all parts beneath the ribs, called hy-

14   RIVERIUS, *op. cit.*, Praxeos lib. Xii, cap. V.

pochondria are affected, yet the spleen most'. In contrast to other authors he places this type of melancholia among the diseases of the spleen. The treatment which he outlined was followed in most universities and is, therefore, presented in some detail. The basic treatment includes the opening of obstructions, correction of the distempers of the body, and discharge of the faulty humor. Medication to strengthen the brain and heart included opium and wine of roses. The treatment should start with a clyster, followed by drinking a potion containing senna, annis seeds and cream of tartar. The following day blood is drawn from the left side of the body. After sufficient purging a bath of warm water with cooling herbs is given and ointment of roses is rubbed on the abdomen to stimulate the liver. The hemorrhoids should be provoked by rubbing the anus with fig leaves or by the application of leeches and a cupping glass. The correction of the distempers of the body is achieved by moistening the body and restraining the violence of the humor, through the administration of baths and fomentations (application of warm wet towels). The discharge of the faulty humors is stimulated by all these means. It might be added that RIVIÈRE disputes the value of mineral waters. He recommends salt or vitriol of iron and oil of sulphur to relieve the obstruction of the liver and spleen.

In a broad discussion of hypochondriacal melancholy, GOTTWALDT (Leyden 1662) states that the existence of black bile cannot be demonstrated and postulates that it is necessary to assume that the cause lies in an inflammation of the blood, the melancholic humor or the bile. Differences in the clinical picture may be caused by disorders in bile, phlegm or acid spirits. These factors may be single or in combination, continuous or intermittent, severe or light. The symptoms described are essentially the same as PLATTER's but with the inclusion of physical illnesses and mental symptoms of depression. He concludes that the internal and proximal causes are the bile, prancreatic juice and phlegm resulting in flatulence, vapors and halitus. The treatment is very difficult and only symptomatic relief is possible, following FELIX PLATTER. GENIUS (Leyden 1669), like GOTTWALDT a pupil of DE LE BOË (SYLVIUS), presents similar ideas. In a later Leyden period, dissertations were under the influence of WILLIS (HANNIEL, Leyden 1677; WALLICH, Leyden 1678). The point made by BATTUS in 1602 is repeated by GENIUS, i.e. that the acid wines from the Rhine and Mosel valley may cause hypochondriacal melancholy. Such intense emotions as terror, fear, worry, or their continuous effect may disturb the animal spirits and result in acrimonious bile. The understanding of the relationship of body and mind became of increasing importance at Leyden under the influence of OOSTERDYCK-SCHACHT and GAUB and is well illustrated by VAN DER HAGHEN (Leyden 1715). He stresses the presence of intense anxiety and its physiological effects. Anger and aggressive furor may have the same psychopathological effects as phrenitis. Such intense emotions are suspected of causing acrimonious bile, leading to retarded motion in the abdomen affecting liver, spleen and resulting in scorbut, cachexia and icterus. The corrupted bile produces sadness 'intercepting the noble relationship of mind and body'.

The widespread influence of WILLIS is seen in the discussion of GERBER (Erfurt 1715). However, he includes symptoms which appear to have been schizophrenic in an interesting review of paranoid depressive symptoms and stresses religious delusions, e.g., having committed an unforgivable sin, of fears of being caught by the devil and being in a frightening, enchanted place. He recommends PLATTER's textbook for further elucidation, and also quotes LOMM's observation of the change of a 'simple and sad melancholia degenerating into a cheerful, as well as furious, excitement'. He then speculates how a connection exists between hilarity, cheerfulness, sadness and an abundance of blood of a fluid and lively consistency.

The impact of HOFER's *De nostalgia* (Basel 1688) was lasting. Still in this century the psychopathologic effect of homesickness has attracted the attention of the clinicians. The author's contribution was often mentioned and a few other dissertations discussed this topic. The physiologic introductory statements of HOFER showed the influence of the presiding professor, the anatomist HARDER (other dissertations which appeared under his guidance were on anatomical and internal medical subjects).

'The essence of the illness is best described by a case presentation. A student from Berne, who studied in Basel, appeared sad, had anxiety and strongly desired to return home. When the symptoms increased in intensity the servants became concerned and a physician was called. The student's health was generally poor and he did not respond to treatment. The physician told him to return home. The patient began to show immediate improvement and was well when he reached Berne.'

Another case mentioned was that of a farm girl who was injured at work and had to be taken to a hospital. She became sad and her only words were 'I want to go home'. When removed to her home she recovered fully in a few days. The author explained the symptoms by continuous vibration of the animal spirits of the middle part of the brain in which traces of the ideas of the homeland have become impressed. Frequent dwelling on this thought impressed it more strongly. He disputes the claim that this disease was endemic in Berne (it might be mentioned that the Swiss soldiers in foreign service during the 16th and 17th centuries frequently suffered from homesickness). The early symptoms of a depression, due to nostalgia, are recognized when a person is tired of learning the foreign language, is easily hurt by jokes, unduly disturbed by little inconveniences, talks frequently and proudly of his homeland and boasts to foreigners about it. When the illness is fully developed the patient loses his thirst and appetite, sleeps poorly, sighs frequently, experiences anxiety and palpitations of the heart, and shows stupidity of the animal spirits. When sent home he improves fast.

HOFER does not emphasize the danger of suicide which preoccupies authors of the present century. In the 19th and 20th centuries the suicidal danger was repeatedly discussed. Cases were published of young nursemaids from rural areas who became homesick and deeply depressed, and in despair killed the child under their care and tried to commit suicide.

The first detailed discussion of *suicide* in medical literature is the dissertation of FRIEDRICH HOFFMANN (Jena 1681). Many previous physicians had briefly mentioned 'violent death to onesself' in the disappointment of love, depression and especially in marked excitement with despair. The means used were drowning, cutting the throat, hanging, poison and self-starvation. No full discussion of suicide was offered by any author. In this dissertation Greek and Roman writers, as well as those of modern times, are well reviewed, including physicians, philosophers and poets. Physicians of the 16th and 17th centuries offered well documented observations (e.g., PLATTER, AMATUS LUSITANUS, TULP, AB HEER). HOFFMANN discusses depression, characterized by sadness and fears, definite or vague illusions and hallucinations, desire for solitude and poor sleep. This description includes depressions of various age groups, as well as schizophrenics with depressive features. He emphasizes this occurrence in senility, as well as in young people. At times his review is rather uncritical, e.g., when he mentions at length the influence of the stars. Dangerous symptoms shown are despair of God's forgiveness, continuous depressions with anxiety and fantastic delusions.

Suicide is stressed in dissertations dealing with the preservation of health, especially of students and scholars (see chapter IX).

3. Schizophrenic Illnesses

Some schizophrenic illnesses are included in melancholia while catatonic reactions are treated as a separate entity (catalepsy) and schizophrenic excitements were considered part of mania. It is difficult to single out schizophrenic symptoms and illnesses in the descriptions of textbooks and among the dissertations. When a case is presented the evaluation of content and affect permits a likely diagnosis, but the absence of a description of behavior and of the course of the illness present considerable difficulty. One is obliged to consider a schizophrenic illness in a case of melancholia when imagination and reasoning are severely and long lastingly damaged and if sadness is not a striking feature. On the other hand, one must keep in mind that nihilistic and grandiose delusions, excitements and deterioration might be related to general paresis and other brain damage which were not as yet recognized.

Some authors use such terms as insania, amentia or desipientia in melancholia with a marked thinking disorder, indicating an illness which corresponds frequently to schizophrenia.

The dissertation of LIDDELL (Helmstadt 1596) is a good example of a discussion of melancholia in which depression receives considerably less attention than the schizophrenic content. The author states:

'That mental disorder is properly called melancholia in which imagination, and sometimes thinking, are affected without fever and furor but with fear and sadness, all without any manifest cause.'

It should be remembered that sadness includes a depressed affect in its narrower sense as well as worrying, unhappiness and the emotion accompanying grief and loneliness.

'The melancholics are affected with the kinds of images when they are awake that come to us when we are dreaming under the influence of alcohol, sex or something similar. And although there is not just one kind of drunkenness, but a kind peculiar to the nature and constitution of each person; some weep, some laugh, some make love, some become angry and kill those whom they meet. This is what happens in melancholia.'

He concludes that timidity is not characteristic of black humor which causes melancholia and mania. Fear and similar reactions come from the heart.

The authors who influenced students were PLATTER[15], who presents clear observations of schizophrenic illness, but under the term of ma-

15   F. PLATTER, op. cit.

nia, and Du Laurens, whose statements of delusions were repeatedly quoted. Platter assigned some of his cases to mania because 'mania and insanity [insania] are such depravations of the mind that their victims imagine, judge and remember many things falsely not only grieving and fearing like the melancholic, but doing everything unreasonably'. His *Observationes* include, therefore, no melancholic patients which might be considered schizophrenic. On the other hand, he states in his textbook that some patients, suffering from melancholia, may be indolent and quiet who do not answer when questioned, or flee the company of men and hide in forests.

> 'This is called lycanthropy after the behavior of wolves.'

Du Laurens[16] includes symptoms in melancholia which Platter assigns to mania. The delusions which he quotes, without emphasis of the affective components, are hypochondriacal of an absurd type, of being transferred into an animal, of being dead and refusing to eat, of being nothing, of being Atlas carrying the world on his shoulders, of being poisoned, of being threatened on the streets and of misinterpreting the behavior of others. It is difficult to evaluate such delusions. At present they would be considered schizophrenic but some of them might also be found in deep depressions of later life. Far-reaching, absurd hypochondriacal delusions are also found more frequently in patients from rural districts. Furthermore, the 16th and 17th centuries were a period of superstition, and the Greek concept of metempsychosis, i.e., that souls go from one body into another, including that of an animal, was accepted also by the sophisticated.

Burckhardt (Basel 1660) quotes Platter's observations and stresses that these patients were depressed, fearful, and had horrible and sad imaginations and estimations of their impressions. In other dissertations one finds interesting case presentations which permit the reader to form his own opinion. Scheffer (Helmstadt 1652) quotes observation 13 (book X) of Forestus. This Louvain student was in the third stage:

> 'He imagined that he had a Bible in his head and consequently kept saying over and over in a Belgian accent: die Bibel is in den Bol – de Bol is in den Bibel, that is, the Bible is the head and the head is the Bible. Finally, he left Louvain, started out for Alemannia and threw himself in a well and drowned.'

The prognosis is more serious when reason is malfunctioning and

16   Du Laurens, *op. cit.* and *Des maladies mélancholiques,* Paris 1620.

especially if the melancholia is accompanied by profound thoughts. It was considered a bad sign if the patient abstained from food.

HEYDENREICH (Jena 1675) discusses:

'A twenty-seven-year-old farmer, of dry and cold temperament, [who] spent his days at rough labor and often spent his nights wide awake. He had thus far drunk very little, and in proportion to the amount of food he consumed, he took a good deal less of secondary beer or water. He often enjoyed the smoke of tobacco. Recently he was frightened by the unexpected sight of a funeral and by a ghost which he said he had seen. He felt swellings of the body along with anxiety and heartburn. He sighed frequently and thought that he was being raised up by his sighs. He neglected food and drink, fled his usual occasions of conversation, was eating his heart out, avoiding men, leading a solitary life, pensively fearful and fearfully pensive. He talked to himself, scowled, burst into tears without any evident reason, and could not sleep. His bowels did not do their duty, and he frequently had acid belches. He argued that he could not be saved. His relatives, who had learned of this from reports of the neighbors, took pity on him and sought advice. In his analysis, HEYDENREICH stresses the "essentially inherent or pathognomic signs: There is mental alienation without fever, since he argues that he cannot be saved, he talks to himself and is engrossed in fear and deep thought. He is pensively fearful and fearfully pensive. There is sadness for no evident reason, and frequent sighs, by which he believes he is lifted up. But this one thing, namely fear and the consequent sadness, is the common sign for all melancholics, as AETIUS says." '

The dissertations include a lengthy explanation of the symptoms based on humoral pathology with emphasis on the affect of fear and sadness, of meditativeness and worry about the solitary life.

MENTZEL (Frankfurt a. O. 1684) gives a history of

'a studious young man, about 23 years of age, who was not accustomed to a balanced diet, and passed from deep sadness into hypochondriacal melancholy. This was in September, 1680. The disease resisted the most careful treatment, although there was partial relief after a while. In the same month in 1681 the disease reappeared. He suffered violent spasms if he ever tried to move in bed. He would look into space and seem to see the head of Medusa [terror] and he would not be able to move his head. Sometimes his feet would be convulsed and he would sprawl on the ground. He would feel pain around the praecordia, and frequent and painful palpitations of the heart. A feeling of warmth in the hypochondrium sometimes preceded intense cold. The bowel was constipated and there were intestinal rumblings. The spleen swelled up and his breathing became difficult. Dreams kept him from getting much sleep: he would often leap out of bed tortured with anxiety. His head was heavy with sleep and he was affected with a total lassitude. He lost his memory almost completely. Sometimes he wept for days, or at least, was saddened without evident cause. Sometimes he was filled with fear and could not be freed from the fear even when persuaded that he was not threatened by anything. When his mind was disturbed he was taken out of himself as if in ecstasy: his face would grow pale; he would become stiff and at times he would speak of arcane things, or rather he would murmur them. When he came to again, he would be unaware of all this. He complained that he sometimes felt pains in the medulla of his bones. His sweat was most rank and his urine various'.

The author, under the influence of DE LE BOË (SYLVIUS), gives quite a different analysis from that of the preceding student (HEYDENREICH). The current interest of the Leyden School[17] seemed to have placed little stress on psychopathological phenomena except when it related to physiological symptoms. This difference between the Dutch medical schools and those of Erfurt and Jena is quite striking and is well illustrated in several dissertations.

BRETSCHNEIDER (Erfurt 1705) described 'a sick man who became melancholic on the occasion of an hypochondriacal disease':

'A certain young man, 24 years old, a student of theology and a master of philosophy, spent the night in his studies as diligently as he could, especially when he thought ahead to the time when he would be leaving school. He spent the whole day at his books, and would leave them as little as he could. He was content with a light lunch and stayed away from his dinner ordinarily. If he felt hungry, he appeased the hunger with bread, butter and cheese. After he did that he got right back to his studies and the books, especially those written about a sudden death which he knew backwards and forwards. He used up much of the night and exhausted both mind and body. Finally he began to feel a weight in his hypochondrium on the left side so heavy that he seemed to be carrying around a rock inside of him.

There came now a continual upset, a great deal of anxiety and a very great sickness of the spirit, resulting in his thinking himself deprived of all comfort, clearly rejected by God, excluded completely from his grace. This he imagined constantly.

His friends worked meanwhile at refreshing his depressed spirit by various talks, and ordered him to hope for better things. But it was a waste of time.'

The previously mentioned VATER (Wittenberg 1680) states that 'by reaction of the spirits the imagination and hence the reason can be so injured that either delirium or melancholy arises'. He defines the delirium as

'mental alienation [desipientia] without fever and furor, but with fear and sadness, and depending on the imaginative and rational faculty. The characteristic symptom, therefore, is not diminution, or abolition, of a function but distortion of

17 WILLIS, op. cit., pass secunda, cap. XI, postulated that melancholia is a complicated distemper of the brain and heart. The heart retards the flow of the blood and the confused animal spirits cause the melancholic condition of the blood.

it, that is, in the false imagination, and also in some of the absurd conclusions of
the reason. Doctors do not call a distorted imagination by itself a delirium, but
require that the reason consent to the distorted material presented by the imagination. A dizzy person whose senses told him that everything was gyrating around
him, but whose mind told him otherwise, could not be called delirious. It sometimes happens to hypochondriacal melancholics that they come in the end to recognize that their fears and sadness are groundless'.

The obvious shortcoming in VATER's definition of a 'sad delirium'
and his summary of the kind of delusions observed is the lack of clear
definition of sadness and its degree. The recognition of the psychopathology of emotions and its significance in psychiatric illnesses was not re-
alized until the 19th century.

In a review of delusions in melancholia, ALBECK (Tübingen 1688)
gives a vivid summary of them which occur in depressive and schizophrenic illnesses:

'They fear jail, torture, the last judgment and eternal condemnation. I don't
know what crimes they think they have committed. They fear that heaven will be
lost, they hate mankind, their friends and turn away from their families. They
have urges to kill those they love dearly and are driving to hurt their spouse.
They blaspheme against God, they are driven to renounce God. They are suspicious and diffident. They have wrong and different types of suspicions. They believe that demons have sent them by the tricks of enemies. They believe that
drugs will poison them. They want to go to far away places and want solitude.
They despise mankind's customs. They hide themselves in corners and hiding
places of their houses ... They are concerned with divine things and imagine talking with God and angels. They think they are talking with the devil and try to
avoid demons.'

It is interesting to note the difference between the knowledge of
clinical observations available at the time of PLATTER († 1614) and DU
LAURENS (1609) and at the end of the 17th century.

Among later dissertations on schizophrenia one might consider
those previously discussed, by GERBER (p. 15) and BÖNNECKEN (p. 4).
Their discussions offer a broad view of melancholia, covering both schizophrenia and depression. SCHULTZ (Frankfurt a. O. 1705) presents the
case of a depressive post-partum psychosis which he contrasts to other
cases of post-partum melancholia with schizophrenic symptoms.

Chapter IV
Mania

Mania, a term used in the sense defined here, was accepted as an entity until the end of the 19th century. Other terms used synonymously were insania, desipientia, delirium, furor, and rabies. It was recognized as an excitement without fever, with anger as the leading emotion and with disturbance of the imaginative and, to a lesser extent, the reasoning functions. Included in the clinical groups which modern psychiatry would recognize are manic and schizophrenic excitements. Catatonic excitements would also be included, but are rarely singled out in literature, and in this publication are referred to in chapter VI. A third group deals with sexual excitements (nymphomania), which attracted considerable attention in the medical literature and is reviewed in the dissertations.

The outstanding authorities cited are PLATTER, SENNERT, and later, WILLIS. The observations referred to are those of VALLERIOLA, FOREST, PLATTER, WEPFER and SCHENCK.

As a basis of this presentation I shall quote a passage from FONTANON[1], who was a professor at Montpellier, and died a few years before PLATTER became a student at that university. His textbook appeared in 1550 and was last reprinted in 1658. In the 1549 edition of his earlier book *On the Cure of Internal Diseases* FONTANON states:

'This disease (mania) occurs when the brain suffers either by itself or by reason of sympathetic reaction. It occurs sometimes solely from the warmer intemperatura of the brain without a harmful humor, and this is like what happens in drunkenness. It occasionally arises from stinging and warm humors, such as yellow bile, attacking the brain and stimulating it along with its membranes. It sometimes even originates in incorrupt blood which may even be temperate but which harms the brain by its quantity alone.'

'Mania is less dangerous if frequent laughter accompanies it, along with behavior which seems ridiculous in the eyes of the onlookers. But, if much yellow bile is mixed with the blood they turn out angry and heedless. But, if it is excessively burned and rendered heavier, there will be brutal madness (furor) and this is the most dangerous mania of all'.

1   FONTANON, *op. cit.*

The statement from PLATTER's textbook[2] gives the following description:

'Mania [mania] and insanity [insania] are such depravations of the mind that their victims imagine, judge, and remember things falsely, not only grieving and fearing like the melancholic, but doing everything unreasonably. Sometimes they are the authors of relatively modest words and deeds which are not accompanied by raving but more frequently, changed into rage, they express their mental impulse in a wild expression and in word and deed. Then they come out with false, obscene and horrible things, exclaim, swear, and with a certain brutal appetite, undertake different things, some of them very unheard of for men under any circumstances, even to the point of bestiality, behaving like animals. Especially do some of them intensely seek sexual satisfaction. I saw this happen to a certain noble matron, who was in every other way most honorable, but who invited by the basest words and gestures men and dogs to have intercourse with her. Add to these, cases where they try to do violence to themselves and to others: they pull their hair out, tear their clothes and sometimes injure their own bodies some way or other by biting. Unless they are tightly bound by bonds and chains, which however they strive with every effort to break, and are kept under guard and locked up (where they will often try as hard as they can to break down doors or escape from their prison by digging), they will attack bystanders, and, like beasts, try to scratch, bite, strangle and kill them.'

PLATTER then continues as follows:

'Some exhibit manic and melancholic symptoms which are sometimes strong, sometimes mild, and perform at the same time things which are praeternatural and (or) monstrous, and openly declare that they are possessed by a demon. On account of that they are called Possessed or Demoniacs. Apart from the depraved actions of mind, as was mentioned, they often remain mute for the longest time, as the demon is wont to make sport of men in remarkable and diverse fashions and to bewitch them. Likewise, they sometimes abstain from food longer than nature would ordinarily tolerate, without, however, any injury. And they sometimes so twist, bend and curve the body that, as I have seen with my own eyes, it could not naturally happen without dislocation of the joints. Or sometimes by prophesying and predicting abstruse things they give divinations and foretell the future, or they understand and speak languages which they had not learned when they were healthy as if the demon were speaking through their mouths.'

In the dissertation of LANNOY (Leyden 1674), who was much influenced by SENNERT's textbook, an attempt is made to offer some order in the symptomatology:

'Mania does not always remain at the same stage or resemble itself but undergoes many differences:

2   PLATTER, *op. cit.*, Praxeos, chapter III.

First, in its magnitude. One variety may be crowded with horrible, violent and truculent symptoms. I remember a case of this here in the hospital in Leyden. This man, who was later cured, stretched and broke metal bonds which for many years had not been used on any of the maniacs. Another variety is mild and is characterized by gentler symptoms like laughter, singing, etc.

Second, in its duration. One variety is continuous and it afflicts without interruption. Another variety is intermittent and its aggravations and paroxysms are felt only at certain times. You will find an example of this latter in FORESTUS, book X, observation 21. This, it can be monthly or annual. Another variety is daily and lasts for many months. Another may be brief and ended or cured in no time.

Third, in its origin. One variety is hereditary, in men whose parents were accustomed to be seized by an insane furor and who themselves are vulnerable to mania. Another is acquired, from internal or external causes.

Fourth, in its outcome. One variety is curable, namely that which is produced by external causes. Another is incurable and can hardly be overcome by any remedies. This kind is often hereditary, as both daily experience and the testimony of experts confirms. The last distinction of causes, by which the disease is distinguished into idiopathic and deuteropathic has, by reason of the many disorders of the brain, no place here. For mania is produced not by vapors or sharp breath but by the very animal spirits secreted in the blood.'

Ten years later, GLÜCK (Leipzig 1685) reformulated the types of mania, grouping them according to 'form, subject, causes and time'. Under form he included [a] delirium with furor and without fever and also hydrophobia, which is characterized by fear of, and aversion to, water and fluids. Under subject he distinguished idiopathic mania, in which the brain and the animal spirits are primarily affected, from sympathetic mania, in which the damage to the spirits comes from the hypochondrium or uterus. The causes may be hereditary or acquired, or demonological or caused by philters. (LANNOY did not mention demonological causes.) Time referred to the course of the illness; i.e., acute or of long duration, recurrent after free intervals or complete recovery.

It is obvious that considerable progress had been made since PLATTER's textbook first appeared in 1602, and reprinted unchanged in 1656, from which edition the above translation has been made.

The theories of mania receive attention in all dissertations following humoral pathology of the 16th century. Among the dissertations I found of interest is the one of HUHN (Helmstadt 1644), who in laborious style, discusses Greek and Roman philosophers, medical and non-medical writers. He then turns to biblical sources, paying special attention to demonology, and reviews some of the thoughts of AVICENNA and the early 16th century. A quite different approach is the dissertation of HORST

(Giessen 1677), who is influenced by VAN HELMONT, M. HOFFMANN, WILLIS and his grandfather, GEORG HORST. He considers the theories from a clinical point of view, and stresses the tragic effect of anger and of violent intensity of love and fear. There are a large number of references to clinical observations in mania, e.g., the causal significance of head injuries. The difficulty for the modern reader is that only the author's name is given, but not the title or year of publication. STANGIUS (Halle 1700) stressed the exogenic factors in mania, including head injury, drugs, poisons from vipers and tarantulas, and rabies. Among the drugs he mentioned belladonna and opium. A more modest, but still valuable, type of dissertation is presented by BUELIUS (Marburg 1680), who applies the theories of DESCARTES, with emphasis on the role of the pineal gland.

These discussions became of greater significance with the increasing preoccupation of the mind–body problem. WINTER (Erfurt 1710) applies the five principles of WILLIS[3] and the concept of fermentation to mania, following closely 'De anima brutorum'. His references to other authors who followed WILLIS (e.g., ROLFINCK, who presided over five dissertations on mania) are valuable. The growing influence of the concept of the soul of WILLIS, over the theory of DESCARTES, appears clearly in psychopathologic dissertations of this period.

In 1734, FISCHER (Halle) expressed it in the following words:

'The soul in all types of manic delirium ... is hurt indirectly and accidentally not per se. For it is a simple being, and a mere thinking substance, according to DESCARTES, can suffer no physical changes ... All changes which sometimes seem to occur because of this profound union with the body are to be attributed to an injury to the body and a disturbance of its motion.'

Review of literature of the clinical aspects of mania is found in the above-mentioned dissertation of HORST and in the contributions of LA GANETTE (Leyden 1723) and FISCHER (Halle 1734). LA GANETTE in the entire dissertation presents the views of outstanding authors of the 17th century on clinical findings and of the Arabian and Renaissance writers on treatment. FISCHER follows a case presentation with a discussion of the works of the Greek and Roman writers. In some dissertations a separation between manic and schizophrenic excitements is attempted, but no clear distinction was possible. In this presentation the dissertations are, therefore, grouped under the two titles, according to which of the two types has been more emphasized or is well represented.

3   WILLIS, *op. cit.*

Reference is made in several dissertations to the relationship of mania and melancholia (e.g., STANGIUS, Halle 1700). There are no clear statements which refer to manic-depressive psychoses. Such observations, as well as the occurrence of schizophrenic melancholia and excitements with affective features or catatonic excitements, no doubt, were made by physicians[4].

An interesting psychological dissertation from Marburg by BOEH-MIUS (1740) should be mentioned because it offers a good understanding of HARTMANN's psychology which is occasionally mentioned in medical dissertations.

Little needs to be added, but a few dissertations may be reviewed briefly. MATTHIS (Strasbourg 1669) stressed: (1) surgical treatment (to evacuate blood and humors from the veins, to remove and divert them from the brain and to cool them); the means recommended are venesection, cupping glass with scarification, leeches and opening of hemorrhoids; (2) pharmaceutical treatment to evacuate bile by giving syrup of manna or succory, rhubarb, senna, extract of hellebore and in clysma, and to cool with borage or bugloss; (3) prescribing a healthy mode of living, which includes avoiding the stirring up of intense emotions.

SCHLAPPERITIUS (Jena 1673) also advised that 'unless there is a tremendous urge, sexual activity should be avoided until mental health returns'. SCHROEDER (Erfurt 1695) recommends physical punishment for furor, but advises against it for the purpose of breaking the patient's silence.

PRINTZ (Jena 1708) follows WILLIS and recommends: (1) control of bile by means of emetics which tame and control the powerful bile, and of purgatives (senna and black hellebore); these medications achieve praecipitation and destroy acidity; (2) the lymph must be restored to its more fluid state by emulsions of white poppy, or peony, by decoctions and potions from them or from bugloss or borage, by a warm bath and by venesection which restrains the bile and makes its control through medications possible; (3) to free the spirits and strengthen them by leeches, by producing blisters on the skin, and by keeping a wound open by a horse hair. WINTER (Erfurt 1710) summarizes: a cure is based on controlling the animal spirits, and to restore them to purity and to healthy motion. This is achieved by taming the wild sulphur of the

---

4   WILLIS in De anima brutorum *(op. cit.)* p. 495, distinguished between continual and intermittent mania. The 'raving excitement' occurs when spirituous saline is changed into acid and sharp.

blood and by tempering the crude lymph. The means to be used are
surgical, pharmaceutical and dietary. The dissertations demonstrate how,
at various times and in different medical schools, theories changed but
not the therapeutic procedures.

1. Manic Excitements

The early dissertation of GUALTHERUS (Marburg 1615) offers as references HIPPOCRATES and GALEN, and stresses the pathognomic symptoms of excandescentia, audacity and ferociousness in the absence of fever. The symptoms are 'sounds in the ears, noises of trumpets and pipes
and complaints about the head and the eyes, staring and observing vision and sparks, terrible insomnia, mumbling indignantly, constantly
concerned and anxious'. The symptoms of the fully developed illness are
the same as in phrenitis (delirious reactions) and melancholia, but much
worse, 'a horrible expression in their eyes, making terrible noises, dancing, yelling and wild attacks on passersby, without fever and fear and
often with poor reasoning'. The effervescent yellow bile is recognized in
the facial expression and the behavior of the patient.

The description is well done and relates to some of the observations
by the older authors which he, however, does not mention. Such an
omission is rather unusual in a dissertation, as the student-writer is
usually emphasizing his critical knowledge of literature. It would be of
interest to know how literature is discussed in other dissertations which
were written under PETRAEUS. One should keep in mind that the clinical
picture of manic excitement may have been considerably influenced by
the customs of the early 17th century, with marked differences in the cities and countrysides of the various regions in Europe.

There are few dissertations which include case records of manic excitements. As has been mentioned, such descriptions are valuable as
seen, e.g., in the presentation by SCHLAPPERITIUS (Jena 1673):

'A man 26 years of age, with a strong bilious condition, given to wild anger
for any cause, who gnashed his teeth if he were irritated, of fleshy build with a
ruddy complexion and red hair, ran the risk of being talked about publicly and
afterward was devoured by grief mixed with anger and vindictiveness, and was a
slave to a young lady day and night. After a while, he turned to another and married her. Scarcely had two months gone by, when, drunk in the company of certain nobility, he was seized by an unusual anger, without any prior fever, cursed
everyone who was dear to him, his parents, his wife and neighbors, and soon dis-

solved in laughter. He was put in chains, but he broke the strongest bonds, felt no cold, had the appetite of a dog, was troubled by sleeplessness, relieved himself in his clothes, and thought everyone was poisoning him. The parents seek help.'

The author reached the diagnosis of mania by the presence of fury, the absence of fever, and by the symptoms described. The primary cause was the brain which is disturbed in its balance of the humors, and secondly, the heart which sends inflamed spirits to the ventricles of the brain. The mediate proximate causes were the predominating hot bilious humors or the hotter and drier blood. The remote mediate causes include, on the natural level, the hot and dry, or bilious, temperament which comes from anger and red hair. On the nonnatural level he mentions his greedy eating and his getting drunk. He also refers to the psychological factors – grief, anger, longing for revenge and love conferred on two persons. It is not believed that the devil played a role because the patient had not spoken in a strange tone. On the other hand, it is believed that a philter was given to the patient because 'the sick man remembers (it) quite well'.

No further observations are given as was customary at the time. One can merely speculate to what extent alcohol played an important role, whether psychodynamic factors were influential, and whether the delusions of being poisoned were significant. At a time when philters were given in food and beverages to induce love for a person, or as a poison, delusions have to be evaluated differently from modern times.

The possibility that various poisons could cause mania had been recognized and was discussed by MATTHIS (Strasbourg 1669). His list is an interesting mixture of good and well-established observations and of folklore and superstition: eating deadly nightshade *(atropa belladonna)* and other poisons (not specified), or the brain of a cat or meat of a dog which had died from rabies, orally consuming menstrual blood, and philters of love or wine curdled by lightening and wolf bites (a frequent cause of rabies). MATTHIS mentions well-known authors as reference for some of the above claims. He differentiates mania along several lines: legitimate and spuria mania, intense, severe and incipient, light mania, idiopathic (located in the brain) and sympathetic (from other organs of the body) mania, and demoniacal mania. As causes he discusses imbalance of the humors, heredity, inflammation of the brain with a high fever, intolerable pain, too high amounts of medicaments (purgatives such as aloe, colocynthus and hellebore; various peppers; catharides), poisons, philters and alcoholism, intense and prolonged emotional reactions, lack of sexual gratification, suppressed evacuation (menses, lochia, hemorrhoids). He mentions further the higher frequency among men, the relationship to dry and warm air, excessive insomnia and vehement body movements (dancing, running, fencing, attacking, yelling and screaming, continuous singing, effusive laughing). Truculent manics were difficult to cure and became chronic. The laughing manic had a better prognosis than the one who was absorbed in thinking. The last chapter of this well-organized dissertation is devoted to surgical, pharmaceutical and hygienic treatment. This dissertation is frequently, and has been for many years, quoted in medical literature. It is one of the best presentations of a manic excitement offering details which are too numerous to be included fully in textbooks.

The description of mania by PRINTZ (Jena 1608), written in an awkward style, shows progress made in clinical observation. He makes a statement, found also in previous publications, that the manic offers the opposite picture of a depressed person. Summarizing his many paragraphs, the following clinical observations are given: the behavior is wild and uncontrolled. The patient may be impudent, merciless, careless in performing tasks, showing a ferocious and menacing expression. He is aggressive, critical, loquacious and verbose. He may be elated, joking and laughing, but easily upset and angry. In fury he smashes objects and uses weapons to hurt and even kill others, but he may also commit suicide. He talks a great deal about his greatness, his sexual desires and love affairs, but is frequently unable to attain orgasm. Such a patient may talk in a foreign tongue which he has not heard before. (This often-quoted phenomenon was usually attributed to a demon's influence, but PRINTZ merely states the fact without interpretation.) The patient has great strength. (In another dissertation it is questioned as to whether this is unusual strength or the behavior of a man who is audacious because he lacks foresight and takes unreasonable chances.) At times patients become untidy, even filthy in appearance, soil the beds and lack shame in their behavior. Patients who are elated are safer to deal with and more amenable to treatment than those who constantly talk of their delusions. Before the onset of the acute excitement, the patient may have studied long nights, or he may have been worried about something, depressed, or indulging in heavy alcoholism. The illness may change from a depression to an excitement, or from an excitement into a delusional picture. The course of mania may be chronic or consist of 'paroxysms with lucid intervals' of varying lengths. Mania has been observed in the first three months of pregnancy. When occurring in puerperium, delusions are frequent. In all excitements, dog bite (rabies was still common) has to be ruled out.

Differential diagnosis advanced as the dissertation of FISCHER (Halle 1734) illustrates. The clinical material includes points which are not essential nor interpreted but seem interesting for the discussion. This type of presentation became increasingly frequent in the publications of the 18th century.

'An honorable man, 44 years old, of a predominantly choleric and drier temperament, thin, and by disposition sensitive, indulged excessively in profound thoughts, particularly in studying at night, eating too little and using tobacco too much. Because of the harm these things did, he became very irritable. When in this violent state of mind, he drank large amounts of brandy. The next night he did not sleep. Arising the morning after, he said absurd things and made unusual gestures, and a little later, in a rage, broke windows with a stick. When his maid appeared he struck at her for no reason. His wife, with the help of the servants, got him to go back to bed. On account of his continual delirium, he had to be restrained just like a maniac to prevent him from throwing himself from the window or hurting someone as he ran about hither and yon. He had no fever, nor was there any suspicion of a hidden illness of the hypochondrium. No hemorrhaging of the hemorrhoids or straining effort to hemorrhage. His bowels were blocked by this raging paroxysm. He had a good appetite and a strong, tense, pulse. There was very little urine and it was thin, sometimes a little reddish, with a sparkling sediment which was a richer shade of the same color. After some days passed without the help of drugs most of the delirium passed.

He remained, however, so extremely sensitive as to sight and hearing, that he was not able to put up with brightly lit things or bright colors such as red, yellow or white. Nor could he bear even slightly loud sounds such as bells ringing, people singing, or going past wearing spurs and leggings, without headache and, as he put it, concussion of the brain, and without a revival and aggravation of the delirium which had not yet been altogether quieted. For this reason he was forced to stay in a place remote from the voices of men and somewhat dark. His wife and friends sought the help of a certain doctor who used hot, bitter, irritating, volatile, purgative and sudorific treatments and led the patient into more trouble. The patient's sleep, which had been short and turbulent, was entirely put to flight by the use of the aforementioned treatments so that the sick man slept scarcely five hours in four days. Fantastic ideas came more frequently and in greater strength and, to the symptoms mentioned before an excessive sense of taste and a tender sense of smell were joined so that anything with a distinct, or volatile, odor, or anything sharp, spicy or salty could not be brought into his presence without pain in the sensory organ and without the above-mentioned mental disturbance.

When these symptoms had kept up for more than a month, and there seemed to be no hope of recovery, they dismissed the quack and consulted another doctor who, after checking the circumstances, wisely figured out that the trouble was primarily spasmodic and essential, judging from the excessive dryness and tightness of the membranes surrounding the nerves of the brain, and of other membranes, and thought that it derived from the bilious bitterness and from a defect of gelatinous fluid. Satisfied with the symptoms, he made use of a bath and a foot-wash prepared from soothing components. He further cared for him at times using a sponge which had been moistened in a soothing potion, then squeezed out a bit and applied to the head where the crown and sagittal sutures meet. He also injected soothing clysters at intervals. Internally he prescribed (a medicine containing many ingredients, including several herbs and components of mercury and sulphur). With these things and a suitable accompanying diet the second doctor diminished the illness a little within a few days, and at the end of nine weeks had wiped it out altogether.'

'Different types of mental problems, or deliria are met with in practice, and they are specifically different in character. Medical schools use this explanation: There are two primary classes, either the acute phrenetic or the chronic melancholico-manic. We dismiss the first kind for the present and leave its treatment to others.'

'Melancholics seek loneliness, burst into tears and sighing without cause. They are tortured by fear, but have no intention of hurting others. They are more fixed in their fantastic ideas, and they cannot be talked out of them by anyone.'

This should not be confused with delirium, phrenitis, paraphrenitis, hydrophobia, lycanthropy, cynanthropy, St. Vitus' Dance, tarantism and amentia.

'Those seized by cynanthropy, or canine rabies, have a severe and malignant fever which was ignited by the poisonous and burning contamination of a dog bite. Because of angina, or an inflammation of the neck, they can force neither solids nor liquids through the esophagus into the stomach cavity, and unless a remedy is found in seven days they die.

Hydrophobia differs from this little, if at all, and neither does lycanthropy except that those who are afflicted with the former flee waters and refuse to swallow any liquid even when they have a great thirst because they regurgitate through the nose all the liquids that they take. Those who suffer from the latter are not only averse to water for the reason mentioned but they also imitate the howling of wolves.'

Some authors are mentioned who attribute this behavior to a demon.

'On the other hand, more recent authors, convinced by stronger reasons and experience, deny these fables any further credence and more correctly classify lycanthropy as a species of melancholy and consider it a result of a depraved imagination. (Cf. WIERUS, On Demon. Prestig, book II, Camerarius, Medit. Hist. Cent. I, chap. 72.)'

'In St. Vitus' Dance and tarantism, or Symbolic disorders [adfectibus symbolicis] there is observed an immense, unheard of and insane desire to dance which in the former St. V. Dance was thought to be generally involuntary resulting from insanity and a peculiar convulsion of the limbs. In the latter, however, it is thought to be caused by a sting through which is communicated the specific, most subtle and most sharp poison of the Apulian tarantula which clings to the membranes and nerves.'

2. Schizophrenic Excitements

In modern psychiatry the evaluation of an excitement with elation and delusional content has remained a difficult diagnostic problem whenever delusions are not in conformity with the elated mood. This problem was solved in previous century by not differentiating between various excitements. A brief attempt to clarify the observations and interpretations offered in a few dissertations is indicated. The observations by PLATTER[5] may serve as the background material with which all the authors were familiar. These observations are also valuable because they indicate the outcome of the illness. The observation (p. 86 of the 1614 edition) of 'mania on account of grief in a woman who was very badly treated by her husband' describes a state in which she was naked, bound with chains, and tearing the mattress on which she was lying into small pieces with her nails. Later, she was bled 70 times in one week and was declared 'cured'. In the mean time, the husband had died and the patient remained well during a second marriage.

Another case (p. 86) was that of a young girl whose family refused to let her marry the man she loved. She developed mania; 'regularly uttering many foul things, she died of the mania'. In another girl (p. 87), the man's family refused permission for marriage. 'She became a manic, and for a long time was bound with chains and shut up in prison. She always called out for him in a loud clamor.' After several years she died of this illness. A man (p. 87) 'was seized by a very severe mania then was, as I saw it, wretchedly detained in a dark prison for forty years, naked and lying on straw because he tore everything else to pieces, taking food from time to time. Finally, he was somehow freed from the mania and walked freely through the city, an old man, white haired and decrepit'. Other observations were quoted by several authors in dissertations.

GLÜCK (Leipzig 1685) describes excitements in which patients are noisy – yelling, insulting their best friends, 'quick to wound and bite,

5   PLATTER, *op. cit.*

and they will, unless you are careful, hurt you with their feet or in any way they can'. 'They do not take care of themselves, eat their feces and rip their clothes. They are awake at night and in a continual turmoil of hallucinations (phantasms) and delusions, disturbed by ghosts and demons. The manics have this in common with the melancholics: wakefulness and a continual jumble of things in the imagination so that the delusions of the manics are more external and the melancholics internal. They exercise great strength and convince themselves they are driven by ghosts and that their insanity is caused by demons.' Some of these thoughts might well have appeared in a psychiatric journal at the beginning of our century.

NICOLAUS (Frankfurt a. O. 1692) urges that

'We should carefully investigate the signs both of oncoming and present mania, so that from them we may come, as it were to the unknown by way of the known. But there are persistent periods of wakefulness, terrible dreams, headaches, unbalanced laughter, irrational anger, continual worry, brightness and shiftiness of the eyes, frequent nocturnal pollutions, ringing in the ears, a quiet and pensive air as if in a state of stupor. There is a tendency to look down on the ground and there is fear and dread. The victims of this foretell the future. Under the force of the disease they fall into various kinds of delirium; some laugh, some are angry, some are sad, some frightened by trivial things. All of them are rash, inclined to hurt their friends or themselves, for they will injure or sometimes even kill their friends. They jump out of windows, tear their clothes, spit out their food, act ferociously and scowl. Their eyes are bloodshot, they are constantly awake, their body gets tougher, their strength becomes unnatural, they are not able to feel cold, their pulses are strong and fast, and if any blood is let, it is raw, thick, warm and black.'

Some of the signs quoted above are found in identical form in the dissertation of MÜLLER (Strasbourg 1654), who also emphasized the statement of Roman writers that excitements with laughter are safer than those with preoccupations.

3. Sexual Excitements

These acute excitements are characterized by an open display of sexual desires and actions with mixed emotions of fear, suspiciousness, elation, anger and transient depressive features. Hallucinations and delirium are infrequent. The terminology varies. Most commonly used in medical literature are: furor uterinus, mania ex utero, hysteromania, furor hysteria or genitalis. Melancholia amatoris is usually a schizophrenic or depressive illness with autistic love or intense preoccupation with a beloved person. The term, 'erotomania', may be used synonymously with 'furor uterinus' or indicate an abnormal intensity of love. Nymphomania indicates that the center of the sexual desires is caused by a disturbance in the clitoris while metromania refers it to the uterus. Some authors apply the term 'satyriasis' to sexual excitements in men, but the term also may be applied to priapism.

Through the writings of ARNOLD OF VILLANOVA[6] and early Renaissance authors, the term 'heroes' which appears in literature as early as the 11th century, was used in the 16th century. To quote PLATTER[7], 'They call this species of dementia by the name of HEROES because it is customarily supposed to befall heroes, or great personages, which reason is rather ill considered since not even the poorest person on earth can dodge Cupid's darts'. SENNERT is more succinct: 'Love in Greek is eros from which the Barbarians name this disorder Heroes, and those afflicted with it Heroticos[8].

Before the 16th century furor uterinus received considerable attention in summarized statements which were concise and apparently based on good clinical observation. Authors of the later centuries, who exerted considerable influence and are given as reference in textbooks and dissertations, are LIÉBAULT (who translated and enlarged the book of MARINELLI, 1562), MERCADO, CASTRO, VARANDAEUS, FERRAND, and PRIMROSE[9]. It is of interest that the authors described this illness in Italy, Northern and Southern France, Spain, Portugal, Germany, and England, i.e., in all European countries.

The case presentations found in the observations of outstanding clinicians and in dissertations permit the recognition of manic and schizophrenic excitements. Other psychopathologic reactions which were included in this group usually belong to the schizophrenic group with a few to manic or depressive reactions.

Observations are offered by PLATTER[7], who distinguished immoderate love which affected the patient to a disturbing degree and interfered

6   ARNOLD OF VILLANOVA, op. cit., De amore heroyco.
7   PLATTER, op. cit. Praxeos, chapter III, animi commotio, and Observationum libri.
8   JOHN LIVINGSTON LOWES, The Loveres Maladye of Hereos, Modern Philogy XI, 4, 1914, traces hereos from the roots of eros and hero.
9   OSKAR DIETHELM, La surexcitation sexuelle, L'Evolution psychiatrique 2, 1966. In this historical and clinical discussion the literature is reviewed.

with leading a normal life from insane love and furor uterinus. In his book, on page 53, he describes a widower who had intense sexual desires for a young relative. On the physician's urging he refrained from telling her, and when she married two years later his love turned into hatred. Another patient (page 54), a married man, revealed his sexual passion to a young servant girl and had a frustraneous love affair with her for a year, suffering from shame, fear, and anxiety. On his physician's advice he helped her to get married by endowing her with a large sum of money, and gradually his love abated. Insane love includes homosexual attachments, of which another author, WEPFER, gives a detailed account. Under the title of furor uterinus, PLATTER describes (page 88) the case of a young widow who soon after her husband's death developed an excitement.

'She not only begged in word and gesture to have intercourse with those who were taking care of her, but also when they did not want to comply with her wishes, she ordered, with great shouting, that English mastiffs (Molossos Anglicos) be brought for the porpose ... she who before was always so devout and chaste had come to this detestable insanity in which she later died.'

The reaction to a love disappointment was described by the often quoted FORESTUS[10], under the title *On Furor from Insane Love.*

'When that handsome young man, the son of JAMES WILLIAM, a brewer was desperately in love with a beautiful girl and could not possess her, he began, as a result of his love, to pass into a wretched furor, so that his parents were obliged to restrain him in chains. He dragged out a long and wretched life in this furor (I had sometimes seen him when I was a boy) perpetually imprisoned, and finally ended his life with insanity.

But another young man of Delph also driven insane by love was lying bound to his bed where he lay neglected and wretched. After six weeks, when he was consumed by his insanity as by a wasting illness, I was summoned. We found him not only insane but so ill treated from the various remedies of attending simpleminded women that I had never seen anything comparable or anything so horrible to describe. They had placed on his bare head a bronze device ordinarily used to warm the bed, so hot when lit that they burned the whole crown of his head.

In the wound that followed the whole pericranium and skin were removed right down to the skull, so that the skull and cranium were stripped bare in an area the size of a crown. They treated the young maniac so wretchedly that for many days altogether he stayed wide awake, and leapt out of his bed so that he had to be confined there by a strong man. We prescribed sedatives for sleep but they scarcely did any good.

10   FORESTUS, *op. cit.* obs. **XXIX.**

When we saw the man altogether neglected, and when we saw that the women were taking such care of his bared head, we ordered rather that a learned and skilled surgeon should be called in to care for the wound since the women had been all along treating him so poorly. We scolded those who were there but accomplished little that was good, and were left grieving that the art of medicine, so excellent and necessary, was held in such disregard by so many, since the sick slip into the hands of the empirics.

Another girl who lay wretchedly imprisoned for many years in St. George's Hospital (in which we have seen such cases kept in chains) had been made mad because of love. She survived for many years and died an old woman. The condition of these poor sufferers is wretched if there is no timely intervention. The examples of this are so many and so manifest, as are the tales of their sad ends, as will be shown in the following SCHOLION.'

SCHOLION: 'It is also a mental illness to be madly in love, and so doctors list love as one of the disorders of the brain which usually after a tragic struggle terminate in mania or melancholy. It is called EROS by the Greeks and AMOR by the Romans. Hence, this disease of love is called *ilisus* by the barbarians and AVICENNA. ARCULANUS called it Divine Passion[11]. The part affected, therefore, is the brain itself as in melancholy or mania, into which diseases it (love) easily passes. The disorder, however, is a symptom of a corrupted imagination, because the mind conceives a beautiful image of a man, or woman, and the boy, or girl, gets such a desire for it, that the love is converted into insanity or furor. This happened in the cases we related. For, as PAULUS says, from a heavy solicitude of mind this furor arises and is contacted from a laborious movement of mind, or the cause of the disease is an image conceived in the mind and the corrupt imagination brought on by love, whence excessive solicitude often burns up the melancholic humor or brings on dry imbalance without the humor, and also brings on less of weight and insanity. And so the first cause is excessive love, and afterwards the humors are burned up, and the conversion to melancholy and insanity takes place. These are the signs of that madness: The eyes are hollow, dry, tearless and blinking; the other parts of the body are uninjured; they are troubled only by this unworthy love. There is no variety of pulse which is particular to lovers but it is similar to that of the disturbed person. When the memory of the love comes back as the result of sight or touch, or the reading of a letter, the mind is struck at once, and so is the pulse, so that it manifests neither its natural evenness nor order.

Lovers are also sad, downcast, sleepless, meditative, full of amorous sighs, pale, forgetful of food, and in danger of dying of the wasting away of desire.

Their sighs are frequent; they mourn, weep, lament, wail, cry out und are overwrought. They are never at peace or repose. They speak foreign and incoherent things. They act silly, are delirious and are insane. They stab, strangle and kill each other. Indeed all these things grow out of black bile, which, we see, quite evidently rises in the course of this disorder. When they are thus excited they recite mournful tragedies, as the poets and tragedians have often shown by many examples.'

11   JOHANNES ARCULANUS, 15th century physician in Padua.

This observation of FORESTUS was given in a detailed translation because it is repeatedly referred to in dissertations. The scholia must be considered outstanding and influenced, no doubt, many generations of students when they wrote a discussion of their observations.

Another author should be mentioned, WEPFER[12], whose observations were quoted. Under insane love, he describes the case of a 45-year-old man who for three years was in love with a 50-year-old minister. The patient refused to accept his love as something perverse to nature. A mutual love developed. 'From this companionship arose the mutual bestowal of reciprocal love.' When the minister died the patient became depressed. On his physician's advice he travelled. In Venice he met 'a nobleman who was the very image of the dead man'. A homosexual relationship developed. The patient 'confessed to his doctor that he was at peace as long as he could behold the picture of the dead man in the face of another living person'. When he had to leave Venice the depression returned.

Under the title of 'erotomania', WEPFER[13] gives the history of a 23-year-old man, who, while visiting Basel, fell in love with a girl who was related to his host. The servants, noticing it, told him that the girl and her family would accept him as a husband. Visiting his parents, he was told that he had become a laughingstock. The patient returned to Basel and, a day after his arrival, developed a manic excitement with a display of anger. After intensive bleeding by phlebotomies his excitement subsided.

VALLERIOLA's[14] patient was a merchant (whose name he avoids mentioning out of professional reserve and prudence) who was

'led from love into insanity. In the daytime, and less frequently at night, he was disturbed by unusual (strange) visions, sometimes aroused to rage and furor and soon afterwards pacified and laughing. At certain moments he insisted that he saw the image of his beloved and fawned on her as if she were present. He complained extravagantly that his beloved did not want to return his love. He spoke of nothing but her and passed his days in gloom and his nights without sleep. He was consumed by sadness and woe, and would have done violence to himself if he had not been prevented by his family. When he had spent six months in this kind of insanity I was summoned and I set out for the place where the sick man was suffering. After much effort, and after many preparations, and with the help of God, I recalled him from this insanity and restored him to an integral mind and to health'.

12 WEPFER, *op. cit.*, obs. 82.
13 WEPFER, *op. cit.*, obs. 83.
14 VALLERIOLA, *op. cit.*, lib. II, obs. VII

The dissertations do not include much case material and it seems indicated, therefore, to give a full translation of LOCHNER's description (Altdorf 1684) which was still quoted in the literature of the 19th century:

'A French girl, both noble and marriageable, was leading an idle life and following a warm diet. After she had had a clandestine love affair with someone below her station, to whom her parents refused to give the nod, she began to be worn out by insomnia. For several days she began to call out loudly, to exhibit the part of her body that distinguishes the sexes, to sing lascivious songs, to look ferociously, and when someone tried to resist the woman in her sexual fury her excitement increased. In fact, if she were not bound with strong chains and held in bed by two or three men, she would conceive a fire in her joints and leap naked from the bed, and if she should encounter some man she would rush fiercely at him and lustfully beg him to perform the rites of Venus with her. She was constantly awake, her eyes glowed, her intentions were bad, her speech was coaxing. Her face was wholly inflamed and swollen. A pungent, sticky mucous humor that almost rotted the bed linen flowed at irregular intervals through the portal of modesty. "And foul breath pouring from black jaws strikes the nostrils with its odor." The pulse was strong, the tongue dried out and there was wasting of the whole body. When a doctor was called, he had the girl confined in a French Medical Torture house [carnificina] where after bloodletting, repeated 30 times in six days, he drew from the girl along with her blood at the same time her insane mind, mad love, dear life.'

In his discussion, LOCHNER explains that the 'boldness and immoderate lust arise from an orgasm of blood and animal spirits'. The brain is affected as can be recognized 'from the injury of the principal functions'. By sympathetic reaction the generative organs are affected, 'which is obvious from the sharp humor flowing from the vagina'.

During the 16th and 17th centuries theses from the medical faculty of Paris attempted to find answers to questions with regard to the sexual functions in women. HUBAULT (Paris 1621) reached the conclusion that sexual excitement is a melancholic affliction, PUYLON (Paris 1630) that insanity comes from uncontrolled love, and MAURIN (Paris 1658) that moderate sexual activity is desirable in melancholia.

The psychological meaning of love, and its psychopathologic changes, received considerable attention in the 17th century. Under the leadership of GREGOR HORST, an interesting group of teaching exercises were published in 1611. HORST presented a lengthy discourse on love as described by poets and philosophers, distinguishing between heavenly and sexual love. Question I, answered by JUNGERMANN (Giessen 1611) referred to treatment of love problems and of psychopathology. Question II (SCHONWALDER) referred to philters, and Question III (BILITZER) to the influence of love on the pulse, a question which had stimulated medical discussion for centuries and which reappeared in the coming centuries in various forms of psychological expressions of sexual unrest. These discussions served as dissertations for obtaining the degree of doctor. The thesis of LEGIER (Paris 1632) and the dissertation of BAJER (Jena 1698) deal with similar problems.

Insane love was described by several frequently quoted authors – PLATTER and WEPFER. PLATTER, in his Observations, refers to the excessive intensity[15] and WEPFER to a homosexual love. BACKHAUS (Jena 1686) offers the definition that 'insane love is a symptom of depraved reason originating in an intense desire to obtain the love object and in the consequent disturbance of the movement of spirits'. His dissertation gives a view of the thinking of the 17th century but does not clarify the issue. KUNADUS (Wittenberg 1681) offers a detailed review of literature. WOLLINIUS (Helmstadt 1661) based his discussion essentially on the observations of VALLERIOLA and FORESTUS. It seems that SENNERT's[16] influence was marked during the whole of the 17th century, and his statement that the primary cause of insane love is 'venereal love which deprives men of reason' was accepted. This love may be 'of any man, or woman, or, in fact, of anything beautiful, or something which seems to be beautiful', resulting in joy which makes them behave in a 'wild and stupid' way if they believe that they can obtain the thing loved, or drives them into grief and sorrow, and even suicide, if they despair of love. NEUHOFF (Erfurt 1711) and FUCHS (Erfurt 1724) review sexual excitements in men considering it mentally the same illness as uterine furor.

HEINTZE (Rostock 1719) offered a group of definitions to bring clarity into the use of diagnostic terms, distinguishing between ardent and insane love (accompanied by depraved phantasies). His classification of 'erotomanic' disorders is quantitative, increasing from the first grade, ardent love, to insane and furious love. He states that in the first grade the patient frequently becomes satisfied, but less gratified in the second grade, and rarely in the third.

Sexual desires and their physiological effect were of considerable interest in the 17th and 18th centuries. Three theses of Paris have the same title and conclusion, but the reading of them reveals differences which are important. The conclusion is that love changes mental ability.

15 PLATTER, *op. cit., observationes.*
16 SENNERT, *op. cit.*

HORNAEUS (Paris 1546) stated that sexual activity can cause as well as cure diseases. YON (Paris 1635) recognizes a drive to love which should not be enforced by drugs. Bad effects of love are the psychopathological reactions described above and they will adversely affect mental ability. Possible damage to the memory resulting from excessive intercourse is mentioned by GILGIUS (Altdorf 1691). Damage to the brain was reviewed at length by BOLLMANN (Marburg 1693) in his dissertation on catalepsy. In contrast to authors of other dissertations, which dealt only with the influence of the uterus, he emphasized the sympathetic reaction of the testicles and brain. Spirits pass from the sperm into the brain. GAILLARD (Paris 1695) attributes the feeling of passion to the mind with all kinds of physical effects. He refers to the hysterical virgin who suffers from states of stupor and fear. Love is basically good; it improves mental ability. BOURDELIN (Paris 1717) states that the body and mind are joined and have a mutual effect on each other. Love has a softening and gentling effect on a man, and passion strengthens the spirits thus improving mental ability. In contrast to the discussions influenced by HORST, the Paris theses do not distinguish sharply between love and sex, using 'amor' in both meanings which makes the understanding of the theses more difficult. There was considered another question which affected psychiatric theory and clinical interpretations up to the present century; i.e., is woman more passionate than man. BUVARD (Paris 1604) and DE QUANTÈAL (Paris 1649) gave an affirmative answer which BUVARD bases on a humoral difference. DE QUANTÉAL mentions that women enjoy greater pleasure during intercourse than men and experience intense orgasm. They are rarely frigid, whereas men are frequently impotent. DE MAGNY (Paris 1720) confirmed that salaciousness increases fertility, and DU CHEMIN (Paris 1576) concluded that unsatisfied sexual desires cause insanity in virgins.

The observation that psychotic illness, depression and schizophrenia, follows disappointments in love has been discussed by several authors. KAMITZER (Erfurt 1705) gives an eloquent presentation of the case of

'a 22-year-old man, of a very wealthy and very old family, a person of outstanding virtues and studiousness, gifted with elegant bodily habits and an excellent disposition who admired a Person, joined to him by blood, with a fervent love. She was a very attractive person from the nobility ... The desire of this unfortunate fellow was a waste of time ... He wore out his body by vain thoughts of love day and night. He was tired but defrauded himself from sweet sleep, and suffered from an astounding sleeplessness. He was next upset by attacks of something resembling melancholy, moving toward amentia, even Mania. He gave himself up totally to these thoughts of love, and wore himself down day and night with a tremendous mental sadness, neglecting needed activities for taking care of himself. Indulging in this bent of mind, he committed serious mistakes in the rules of good eating. As a result he developed palpitations of the heart, extraordinary trembling of the body, an unusual excitement in his limbs, and, in addition, tightness around the chest, more and more often. He also got a kind of fainting attack, accompanied by dizziness and weak vision.'

Based on the observations of SCHENCK[17], and VALLERIOLA[18], there are also dissertations discussing psychotic illnesses which are caused by excessive sexual activity. SCHENCK mentioned a middle-aged married man who 'indulged so freely in sexual activities and was so dried out that many days later he was struck by a violent furor'. Drugs given as philters which cause excessive sexual desire may lead to philtromania, as is frequently mentioned in literature. SCHONWALDER (Giessen 1611) discussed the philters, and L'ESPICIER (Paris 1636) emphasized that spicy food in the form of purslane stimulates sexual desire. LEHMANN (Erfurt 1715) gives a list of drugs which were considered sexual stimulants, among them hippomanus which, according to some, was from a plant and, according to others, from the genital mucous of a mare or from animal testicles. Philters contained such plants as *Atropa mandragora*, nightshade and antirrhinum (speedwell). Spicy food and drink were also considered aphrodisiacs, as well as warm and dry air.

The pale facies of young girls of marriageable age who were in love, their lassitude, poor appetite and loss of weight attracted the interest of physicians of the 17th century. The dissertations on this febris amatoria which in the 19th century was called chlorosis, are of minor psychiatric interest.

It is difficult to evaluate the cultural factors which, in this period, affected sexual psychopathology in women, especially in the unmarried. The disease of virgins of marriageable age and of widows, the furor uterinus, was neither common nor rare. The teaching of AVICENNA, explaining sexual excitement by the suppression of menses, was accepted by many until the middle of the 18th century. SENNERT maintained that an important cause was the influence of the demon. The writings of LEMNIUS[19], emphasized the sexual non-restraint of the lower social

17   SCHENCK, *op. cit.*, de mania, obs. III.
18   VALLERIOLA, *op. cit.*
19   LEMNIUS, *op. cit.*

classes in Flanders, a fact which is depicted in Flemish paintings of the 16th and 17th centuries. From literature one obtains the impression that there was a great deal of debauchery in England and in the countries on the continent in the 17th century. The medical dissertations do not offer elucidation of the cultural factors, nor do the writings of leading physicians.

The treatment of furor uterinus is the same as in the other types of mania (BACKHAUS, Jena 1686; BIELER, Jena 1717). Bleeding by venesection, and other types, is considered important, especially when menstruation has ceased. The avoidance of what was considered a sexually stimulating diet was stressed, as well as the drugs which were used as philters (LEHMANN, Erfurt 1715). Some authors stressed that too high amounts of opium may lead to excitement. Psychotherapy was stressed in several dissertations, not only the removal of the unobtainable love object, avoidance of exciting literature and music, and distraction by mental and physical activity. The need for modification of the mode of living should be considered individually. There are also indications in some dissertations that an understanding of the patient's sexual problems and of his life situations was necessary for adjustment. The indication, or contraindication, of sexual intercourse and the use of alcoholic beverages was evaluated (MAURIN, Paris 1658; SCHLAPPERITIUS, Jena 1673).

The prognosis was always considered serious but little is known about the outcome except in patients who developed a deteriorating schizophrenia. (In modern psychiatry the therapeutic results are good except in a few cases where sexual excitement was only a phase in a schizophrenic deteriorating illness[20]).

20   DIETHELM, *ibid.*

Chapter V
Catalepsy and Ecstasy

Symptoms of catalepsy were well described by Greek writers and GALEN's case was still quoted in the 18th century. With the publication of additional cases in the 16th, 17th and 18th centuries more symptoms were added and a clearer distinction between catalepsy and coma became possible. The clinical significance of the cataleptic symptoms remained more or less obscure until the 19th century when the study of the course of the illness led to further clarification and to the concept of catatonia. The occurrence of catalepsy in hysterical reactions was discussed in the 17th century and its relationship to suggestion in the 18th century. From the Greeks to modern times the problem of ecstasy, the differentiation between religious and pathological ecstasy, its relationship to hysteria, schizophrenia, epilepsy and to anxiety has remained a challenging problem. All of these thoughts appeared at various times and in varying degrees of clarity in the observations and discussions presented in medical dissertations.

The term used was 'catalepsis' (meaning to be seized) and less frequently its Latin translation of 'prehensio', 'deprehensio' or 'detention'. Referring to the change in humors and vapors which were claimed to cause these symptoms some authors spoke of 'congelatio', i.e. the congealing, or freezing, of the humors and of the muscles.

The textbook of RONDELET[1] is frequently quoted in literature concerning catalepsy. The following quotations will illustrate the discussion of this author who influenced the medical students.

'*Catalepsis* is a certain seizing of soul and body in which those who are stricken remain in the postion they were in when seized. The mind and all the senses are in its grip and every one of their faculties seem to be consumed. All of a sudden they become mute, but they do not fall down. They remain standing if they were standing and sitting if they were seated. Their eyes are open if they were open before. Hence, the popular opinion is that they do not feel pain, that

---

1   RONDELET, *op. cit.*, chapter 20.

they are the living dead, or that they are carried away, as the saying goes. In that disorder everything is rigid ...'

'The sick are mentally and physically in the grip of the disease so that they have fixed eyes and unmoving eyelids, and sometimes have them open and blink or look intently so that even if someone stretched out his hand toward their eyes they would not close them. Some say that they have perpetually opened eyes which are held so because of the dryness of their eye muscles. Just as in Lethargus and Carus they close when the humor is dissolved. Some are deprived of voice and sensation neither hearing nor answering. But, sometimes they move their hands to their heads, their eyes and their noses like someone plucking at something. They do this without feeling it. Sometimes they speak a bit ...'

'True catalepsy is when from the injury of its actions no one doubts that the brain is affected, especially in its posterior parts.'

'Catalepsy in general is an injury to the principal animal functions and, in particular, to the paralyzed, or abolished imagination. All the remaining functions are somehow injured in it. Respiration, however, survives while the spirits remain uninjured and minister to respiration as a vital necessity. Others feel indeed that the cataleptics are deprived of all motion, but not of all sensation, neither exterior nor interior, because they see, hear and sometimes reason and remember as GALEN teaches in his scholastic history – if they have fallen into this evil as a result of the brain being cooled and dried out from too much study. This symptom follows a cold and dry imbalance ... Catalepsis is produced from a melancholic juice, or vapor, obscuring the back part of the brain. There is another kind of catalepsy which Aetius thinks is produced by copious blood distending the veins and arteries by its mass and keeping them tight just as the plenitude of humors contracts the nerves in a convulsion and holds them that way ... Some authors say that both catalepsies occur the same way as apoplexy, namely as a result of the substance of the brain being irrigated by a melancholic humor or by blood. But, it is doubtful whether it can become cold and dry as the result of imbalance alone as GALEN thought.'

Another author of considerable influence, HERCULES SAXONIA[2] states:

'When struck the muscles, and with it the posture, remain [fixed]. The patient is insensible but vision, hearing and sensus communis remain intact but in severe cases there may be paralysis of imagination.'

The observations of GALEN[3] and FERNEL were known to every student and teacher and they are, therefore, given in translation. GALEN describes

'A certain fellow student, who had worn himself out by steady application to his studies, was seized by this disease and lay as if he were wood, stretched out

---

2   HERCULES SAXONIA, *op. cit.* de melancholia and in *Prognoseon practicarum,* libri duo, Frankfurt 1610, p. 57.
3   GALEN, *op. cit.*

stiff and unbending. He gave the impression that with his eyes open he was looking at us; he did not even blink, but nonetheless he did not say anything to us. He
said [later] that he heard us at the time we were speaking, not always clearly. but
there were things which he recalled. He said that he saw everyone who was present so that he was able to describe some of their actions which he had observed,
but he could neither speak nor move any member.'

FERNEL's[4] cases have led to much discussion in literature. His case
2 was accepted as the paradigm of catalepsy:

'A second [person] I saw lying like a dead man; he neither perceived nor
heard and, when pricked with a pin, did not feel anything. His breathing, however, was easy and whatever was put in his mouth he promptly swallowed. Lifted
off his bed he stood by himself and when given a push he fell down. Whenever
his arm, leg or hand was bent there it remained fixed and stable. You would say
that he was imitating a ghost or a statue that had cunningly learned to walk.'

The diagnosis of the first case (see below) which FERNEL also considered catalepsy was questioned by later authors including respondents in
their dissertations. With the passing of time an increasing number of authors made the diagnosis of coma, or apoplexy, based on the following
description of FERNEL:

'One person was suddenly seized with catalepsy while he was poring over
books and papers so that he stiffened in a seated position, fingers clamped on his
pen, eyes staring at his books as if he were studying them until he was called and
given a shove. Then he was seen to lack all sensation and motion.'

Among the textbooks of the early 17th century, that of SENNERT[5] is
usually referred to in dissertations. His definition adds little that is new
except for a differentiation in degree.

'The malady attacks a man suddenly, and no matter what the man is doing –
awake, drowsy, drinking, eating, writing, reading, he stays that way as if he were
frozen. The sick person keeps his eyes open, fixed and motionless, the eyelids rigid, open even when threatened. In the senses, though, there is a difference in some
[patients]. Those who really have genuine catalepsy, hear nothing, and see nothing, although the eyes are open because the mind is paying no attention. Some
hear and see, but can say nothing. Some seem to move a hand. Some people, if
they are pushed, walk, but remain like statues. Some seem to be dreaming. Respiration continues, but at intervals they heave a great sigh. The pulse is lethargic; not
so much slow and soft, but very regular. The bowel movements and urine are retained, the expelling force being dulled and not responsive to the pressure of the
excrement.'

'But sometimes, when the problem is less powerful, the sick persons hear,
see, imagine and remember something they hear said by bystanders, and after-

4   FERNEL, *op. cit.*, lib. V, cap. II, De lethargo.
5   SENNERT, *op. cit.*, lib. II, part. III, sect. I, cap. IX.

wards recall it, but they remain without a voice and the sense of touch just as GALENUS told of his fellow student.'

While previous authors had stated that a combination of catalepsy and coma may occur these two conditions were separated in the early 17th century. The dramatic cataleptic symptoms, which had attracted attention, now also became connected with prolonged stupor in which the eyes were kept open. SENNERT also emphasized that catalepsy was a dangerous illness, and unless it ends quickly the patient dies from general weakness or through suffocation because the immobility prevents movement of the chest and breathing becomes suppressed.

Catalepsy was rarely seen by physicians, and undoubtedly students were urged to discuss this interesting and puzzling clinical problem in their dissertations and to present new case material. Even so, I found only four dissertations which include case descriptions but they are valuable because few detailed observations are found in medical literature. Besides GALEN and FERNEL the authors most ferquently quoted were BENEVIENI, AMATUS LUSITANUS, TULPIUS, VALLERIOLA, PLATTER, HORST and WEPFER[6].

KHONN (Strasbourg 1662) reviews the literature well and applies his knowledge to a discussion of diagnoses and treatment. He concludes that cataleptics are deprived of intellect, sensation and motion but that not all patients are affected in the same way. He mentions that some patients seem to have visions or dreams, and that some feel pain. His differential diagnostic discussion is clear and defines well the essential differences between catalepsy and apoplexy, epilepsy, lethargy (sopor), coma and fainting. Stupor vigilans is accepted as part of catalepsy.

SCHLEIERMACHER (Giessen 1695) offers a valuable discussion of definitions as found in the literature of the classical writers and those of the 16th and 17th centuries, with emphasis on published observations.

Theoretical discussions follow the thinking of the authors who have been quoted previously adjusting it to changes in humoral pathology (e.g., RONDELET and SENNERT). MANGOLDT (Basel 1673) states:

'The cause of this symptom is a disease of cold and hot imbalance depending on melancholic humors and vapors endowed with the power to direct spirits, blocking up the parts of the brain, not only qualitatively but quantitatively harmful to the nervous system. Thus it happens that not only the animal spirits but, also, the brain is frozen (congealed) and dried up which brings the tension and rigidity of nerves.'

6   Op. cit., observationes.

After a description of the disease's symptoms, DE MAN (Leyden 1671) wrote:

'We will weigh again the opinions of GALEN and SENNERT which many are precipitate to depart from, for I would think it a shame to divorce ourselves vainly from the heritage of antiquity.'

He then gives several brief observations and writes:

'In these and other cases (many of which can be found in the histories of SCHENCK, RONDELET, TULPIUS and others[7] people who have recovered from this disease report that sensation sometimes remained with them.'

He then refutes GALEN's theory that the constriction is due to cold of the spirits or humors and SENNERT's coagulation from a vapor. A constant fixed position of the members is possible only if the influx of spirits into the brain continues.

'One must conclude that those [spirits] which boil up to the brain fresh from the heart are more immune to constriction than the others.'

Of several dissertations of this period (DE GRAEF, Leyden 1676; WENDIUS, Erfurt 1692; RÖSER, Rinteln 1692; BOLLMANN, Marburg 1693; MUYS, Utrecht 1701) ALBINUS (Leyden 1676) deserves to be quoted expressing well the teaching and thinking of the influential Leyden school. A brief presentation of the various definitions is concluded by DESCARTES' warning:

'We worry more about words than we do about things.'

He then offers a concise but detailed review of symptoms as given by FORESTUS, GALEN, PLATTER and FERNEL, and continues:

'The philosophers and doctors of every age have tried to explain the phenomena of motion and sense, and those things which happen in the temple of the body without the attention of the mind, but when they rush with unwashed hands, as the saying goes, wrapped in their prejudiced feelings, precipitately into the sacred places of nature, the result is that they have left us a miserably weakened and defiled science of nature. Lest they should seem ignorant of the things of which they actually are ignorant, they have invented for themselves a bunch of natural and accidental potencies and have subdivided them into vegetative, sensitive, appetitive, locomotive and rational ... Physicians, however, were patrons and authors of the terms, nutrition, growth, reproduction and the things that are of service to them (D. SENNERT). So, in order to get an explanation for the present from these and similar principles, they have so wretchedly tortured themselves and have presented such implausible connections between causes and effects that it is

7   Op. cit.

apparent enough that they are satisfied to spread some kind of veil over their ignorance ...'

'Since we have stripped man of his humanity by splitting him up in parts, we
see those things which cannot be connected nevertheless here united: that which is
nowhere we will see circumscribed by environment; "thinking" and "reaching out"
act on, and are acted on by, each other. Certain ideas follow certain movements;
from these movements or from actions and experiences the mind forms judgments,
and judgments need the help of the body. What is the connection? How are they
joined? The administration of a state by a prince is proof that at the sight of his
name and tokens of his rank whole armies move, and yet there is no connection
between the said effect and the tokens except the good pleasure of the prince and
the custom of the kingdom. There is, therefore, some "Superior Being" at whose
pleasure, after thought, animal spirits, just like a group of soldiers or distinct
companies of them, are put into this part or that part of the body, and vice versa,
as if they were so many guards put on duty.'

'And although the mind is totally united to the body, insofar as the mutual
relationship of the organs makes them indivisible, there are many things which
take place in it which the mind does not pay attention to or which it does not no-
tice even if it does pay attention. As result, the things which are automatic and
as mechanical as if the soul were not in the body (as seems to be the case with
beasts) ought to be explained, since the old authorities make many mistakes here.
Such are chylification, circulation of the blood, nutrition, respiration and digestion, the last two of which DESCARTES, as usual, very accurately explains in *De
Homine.*'

'It will not be easy to explain the phenomenon that the patients stay fixed in
one position, their limbs motionless, since the mind, intent on performing its functions, directs the spirits as if they were so many rivers flowing constantly from
living springs, as the stable pulse indicates, to one or another center of circulating
humors that it may take away the balance. If, by chance, the blood vessels of the
choroidal plexus are excessively opened so that the phlegmatic humors pour out,
which reside in the pineal gland or thereabouts, to produce immobility, then the
members stay in the position they were in when the gland so determined the
movement of the spirits, and as long as it stays in that position, spirits necessarily
flow in the same way, and so, whether the patient lies with eyes closed, or stands
staring, he stays in the position he was in when he became cataleptic.'

ALBINUS then discussed the anatomical studies of the brain by BAR-
THOLINUS, WILLIS and DRELINCURTIUS, and possible localization of catalepsy in the brain, and briefly reviewed the treatment. This dissertation
was widely read and was reprinted in 1690 in Frankfurt a. O. where AL-
BINUS was professor of anatomy and medicine.

In 1692, FRIEDRICH HOFFMANN published his *De affectu cataleptico*[8], addressed as an epistola to G. W. WEDEL which greatly influenced
succeeding dissertations on this topic. His detailed case history, howev-

8   FRIEDRICH HOFFMANN, *De affectu cataleptico,* Frankfurt 1692.

er, is not characteristic of a catatonic illness. The young woman experienced brief cataleptic states with exstasy, part of a hysterical reaction. The author reviews the pertinent literature and explains catalepsy by 'blockage of the corpus callosum which happens by stagnation and extravasation of the blood or fluid in the middle of the brain'. See HOLLERIUS (liber 1 – de morb. intern.) and SCHENCK (liber 1, obs. 2) for the reasons why the major veins of the head of those who died of catalepsy were found, on dissection, to be filled with raw and hardened blood, and likewise their brain filled with a serum-like material. From this it is also evident why a large nosebleed sometimes frees one of catalepsy. See AETIUS. '... Hence, it is also clear why catalepsy sometimes follows the suppression of the customary and ordinary outpourings of blood.'

A good brief presentation of the clinical picture is found in a dissertation by BLOCHMANN (Halle 1708) which includes chapters on apoplexy, paralysis, sleep, catalepsy and vertigo. MÜLLER (Jena 1741) presents in full the case which SENNERT published in 1654 (see below) and a brief summary of a patient seen by his teacher, TEICHMEYER. He then gives a detailed and careful account of his own observations: an 18-year-old man of noble birth, whose mother had been melancholic all her life, had been greatly concerned about marked scars from small-pox which he acquired in early life. He was studious, but in the summer (August) he was much distressed by a toothache and swelling of his cheek. His interest turned to the study of philosophy and later he wished to attend performances of tragedies and comedies. Frustrated in his desire to become an actor he appeared depressed and preoccupied. In September he was worried about the prolapse of his anus (his physician found hemorrhoids), complained about feeling weak and was convinced of his imminent death. He ate little lest his bowels become obstructed. After nights of poor sleep he was fearful, trembling, weeping and praying. He avoided people and prepared himself for his death. In October he appeared stupid with intervals in which he answered relevantly and at another moment became silent. At this period his constipation cleared up and he began to eat large amounts of food. This was soon followed by taking only large amounts of tea and a light diet. The patient now became stuporous and a phlebotomy was considered.

'Therefore, one October morning when he appeared rather happy, a vein in his foot was opened. The blood, which was not especially dark or thick, but was on the red side, was taken through a small opening. He talked after the incision was made, but mostly of melancholic subjects. He released urine without being aware of it. The bowel was not responsive, but was stimulated for a week by clysters ... The remedies either did nothing or aggravated the worst features of the disease: covered with sweat he would often lie for a long time in a wakeful coma; the pupils of his unmoving eyes widened and his limbs were motionless. The urine was often stopped up for 36 hours at a time and would then be released violently and abundantly. The doctor's orders then were to make haste slowly, something to be recommended when dealing with an independent youth. The urine which was drawn off in a glass was thin, grainy and watery, and then cloudy. The symptoms were sudden severe coughing, sweats, purplish itchy skin eruptions which caused scratching, none of which posed a real danger to health. When he was out of bed he suffered light convulsions, trembling of the lower lip, and of the eyelids, heat and intense sweating. A strong pulse would precede the first paroxysms. There was not complete apyrexia so to speak, for there was no manifest fever, but just a slight remission. He had been considered for several days to be speechless, but then he began to recite prayers and to read out of a book which had been placed in front of him. Soon his voice stopped again and he would not continue either in response to prayers or violence.' ...

'In the months of November and December, the nearer it got to the winter solstice, his silence was more constant than that of PYTHAGORAS and became a source of wonder to everyone. A hundred times over it was said that he was dead. Some said that it was just subbornness but they had not seen how totally emaciated he was, with his skin just hanging to his bones and the itching eruptions in the area of the *os sacrum*. His buttocks were chafed, and there was a small gangrenous place. Sometimes people would shout into the sick man's ears, assuming that since he did not say anything he must be deaf. But he would then put up his hands against the person shouting which showed that he was neither deaf nor suffering from blockage of the ears; sometimes, in fact, he would grow quite angry. The same sluggishness of the bowel continued. Except for one day when its weight was astronomical, the urine was not usually emitted or was emitted only with a violent effort of the expelling bladder. Some slight alacrity seemed to be restored but now the sick man betrayed restlessness and unwillingness to go to bed even though he would stagger when leaving it. The aggravation and continuation of this behavior seemed to threaten a forthcoming change of the disease into St. Vitus Dance. An almost canine hunger now began to appear more and more. The bowel was sometimes obstructed for twelve days; when all other hope proved vain, it was finally opened by the usual dose of senna. It was then that the sick man made the greatest efforts. He seemed to be of sound mind, and free will seemed to be restored to him. Nonetheless he still did not talk. When the bowel was not released he lay in an even greater stupor, with a red face and one eye inflamed and tears dropping from his eyes. With the greatest difficulty he was induced to try more remedies. When the senna did not work, the unfailing colocynth clyster was used.'

The physicians decided that the disease was localized in the common sensorium because the medulla is the seat of will, intellect and attention.

'After the new year, as time went on he seemed to be improving in his senses and in his general strength. While sleeping he would move his hands and gnash his teeth. He would use his feet at first merely to stand up, but then during February to walk, although he was very slow at it. The only reason that he walked at all was that he saw food placed in some part of the room. For months he had exhibited such sluggishness of his members that his arm, statue-like, kept for a long time the same curvature into which someone had moved it. A more auspicious sign was that when he was placed on the latrine, he straightaway released urine. The bowel, however, continued to be slow, so that half an ounce of senna leaves would produce merely urine. His face was no longer sad or darkly melancholic, but his expression was foolish or fretful with interruptions of smiles.'

...

'He began to utter a few words after having been for three months silent as a fish, but these were in a very low voice and were directed only to his intimates, his little brother or his sister. He was in a conspicuously bad mood, but in March he was continually smiling or drawing up his cheeks like a monkey, and continually drooling. He walked slowly like a ghost. He suffered from a general weakness, which, however, seemed to improve. This continued into April and was accompanied by insatiable hunger so that once when he was shown a bouquet of fresh flowers, he snatched them up to his mouth and devoured them like an Assyrian cow. Likewise he tried to chew up tallow candles when he had a chance.'

... 'That longed for and happy day, Sunday, May 7, dawned. At this time, after days of warm spring sunshine, the earth was gripped by a new frost and there seemed to be a threat of winter beginning all over again. There continued the same bad mood, stupid dullness, drooling, slow gait, consumptive look, absence of activity, perpetual voracity, quest for food, abhorrence of drink, and almost complete silence, but he would direct a fatuous smile, or a stiff or yokel's expression toward those who spoke with him. This is the condition that he was in before noon. But after noon – behold! He was seized by a paroxysm of intermittent fever, was pained in the area around the heart and began to vomit. His joints were affected, he shuddered and suffered chills. His attendants took these convulsions to be signs that his end was near. He, on the other hand, when visited by the doctor, understood that all were of good cheer and he announced that the happy end of all his ills was near. When orders or questions were proposed to the sick man, he would offer some obscure statement with a faltering tongue and laugh like HERACLITUS but blandly. This was followed by heat, sweating and a quiet night. The next day, the sick man, in perfectly sound mind, called his nurse because of the unheard of event of his having dirtied his bed with urine and excrement, and he asked for clean bedding. Then he continued, showing that he knew that the day was Sunday, and he asked to have the right clothes brought to him. So from a mute, dirty, stupid, foulsmelling and ghost-like figure he became in an instant affable, good-natured, likeable, tidy, bright-complexioned, vivacious.' ...

'This was not the absolute end of his ills, for having been weak before, he quickly became athletic, fat – in fact, his weight doubled – and his balance was once again disturbed but for the opposite reason. He was sound in memory and judgment. He was not only physically healthy but strong as a bull. His will, however, was wandering, inconstant and sick now, so that you would have called it a case of that mental lapse or wandering melancholy which the Arabs call Kutubuth and which was described by SENNERT and BELLINI.'

The patient finally recovered from this illness which lasted a year. As far as it is known this is the first case of catatonia in medical literature which is described in full. As the treatment of catalepsy is discussed below (p. 23), MÜLLER's therapeutic procedures, which followed BOERHAAVE's principles, are omitted from this presentation.

The term 'melancholia attonita' was used by SENNERT[9] when he discussed

'this rare disorder [which] was observed by the illustrious Doctor JACOBUS JANUS ... in 1630 in a man who for thirty years or more had been pastor of a certain church. He was of a melancholic temperament, and in springtime began to suffer from melancholy. He [at once] became sadder, but did not behave in an absurd fashion. Nonetheless, he was troubled, as it were, by certain temptations and because of sins [which he had] committed in his youth. They were not serious, [but] being altogether light, but he had persuaded himself that he could not be [able to be] restored to God's grace, and he considered himself unworthy to exercise the ministry of the church. So, like a man in despair, he passed not only the whole spring, but also the whole summer this way, and from time to time tried to lay violent hands on himself or his wife. He seemed to act, as it were, in a paroxysm. In the autumn, as the excited activity began to let up, he became unnaturally sad, kept silent, and only uttered frequent sighs. Finally, he seemed willing to pay attention to his friends around him who were seeking to soothe his misery with various consolations. He could not be brought to the point of giving an answer, although he was plied with various propositions and questions. Sometimes he would utter one expression: "Oh, God!" Except for this, it was impossible to get a single word out of him for several weeks, even though he was frequently questioned and admonished to speak. Meanwhile, he would sleep at night and awake in the morning only to lie motionless in bed, like a man in deep thought. His wife lifted him up and got him dressed. Once dressed, he stood like a statue, holding his hand to his head and temples, as the unnaturally sad are accustomed to do. He would sigh, and, if given a shove or led by the hand, he would walk. He would sit down when led to a seat or bench. He would sit the table and, when his wife put food in his mouth, he would eat it; and when a cup was placed to his mouth, he would, if told to, take hold of it and drink from it. This disorder lasted throughout the autumn. In the middle of winter it began to diminish, so that he was restored to his ecclesiastical functions and performed them. He is still in charge of the church, but sadder, because he has been naturally melancholic for a long time.'

9   SENNERT, *op. cit.,* and JOH. JAC. MULLER, *diss. cit.*

In the early 18th century the term, melancholia attonita, was used by BELLINI[10] in his widely read textbook. Catatonia replaced the term (KAHLBAUM, 1874), but melancholia attonita was still used in American literature at the end of the 19th century. The term led to considerable confusion because melancholia was considered synonymous with depression, and melancholia attonita was distinguished from catatonia.

MÜLLER called the illness the scholars' disease (morbum litteratorum) since his patient was a student. SENNERT's patient was a theologian. A third case, cared for by B. WEDEL, was studious as was also a patient who had been observed by the presiding professor, TEICHMEYER.

In his Observations, NICOLAUS TULPIUS[11] described the case of a young Englishman who, after having been rejected in a proposal of marriage, developed a cataleptic state. A similar case is found in the dissertation of SCHILLING (Giessen 1676). This 27-year-old man had fallen in love with a beautiful girl.

'When the girl's parents refused him, he was so struck by this unexpected refusal and its meaning, that he became totally immobile and, as it were, frozen and stiffened ... He thus sat on his chair for a whole day ... When the astonished mother came she tried in various ways to arouse him but all was in vain. Finally she exclaimed in a loud voice that she hoped he would have his wish and have the girl he desired. Behold, her son immediately jumped off the chair and came to as if awakening from a sound sleep.'

SCHILLING's discussion is concerned with the diagnostic clarification and the treatment, and not with evaluation of the role which the psychological factors played.

The relationship of catalepsy and epilepsy interested several authors. In the spring of 1685, WEPFER[12] saw a 15-year-old girl who had suffered from convulsions since the age of five. Now, however, her seizures changed:

'Whatever bodily position she was in, whether standing or sitting, and whatever place she was in, her eyes became fixed in a stare, her lips grew livid and were drawn into her mouth, and she sometimes sighed and made the most remarkable gestures ... 'In August the paroxysm occurred once a day for three days. On the thirteenth and fourteenth it attacked her twice. The duration of the attacks is short, scarcely seven or eight minutes, never a quarter of an hour. Often they are much shorter. After the paroxysm had passed away, she would not be aware of anything, except that she would know that she was no longer in the same place

10   LAURENTIUS BELLINI, *Opera omnia*, Venice 1732.
11   TULPIUS, *op. cit.*, lib. I, cap. XXII.
12   WEPFER, *op. cit.*, obs. CXXI.

or working at the same task as before her attack, and she would wonder how she got from one place to the other.'

WEPFER concludes that

'The disorder seems to be some kind of catalepsy for her body usually stays in the same position that it was in during the attack. It differs, however, in that she sometimes speaks, does what she is told, walks, brings things that she has been sent for, answers questions sometimes appropriately, sometimes deliriously, sometimes gestures with her hands, etc. In that she is very close to catalepsy, in that she is unaware of everything done or said by herself and by those standing around.'

'It is doubtful whether there is anything convulsive along with this, for the gaze of the eyes is fixed but the eyes are not rolled backward, the lips are drawn in, but the teeth are not clamped shut, the face and lips grow livid, the pulse becomes frequent and fast but the respiration remains the same.'

The dissertation of GLOCK (Tübingen 1690) does not add much to the observation and discussion of WEPFER. He describes cataleptic epilepsy in the following way:

'Since the limbs of the epileptic remain motionless and still during or after the paroxysm, he is to be described as suffering from catalepsy ... In the disorder I am discussing the parts of the body, sometimes the strongest, sometimes any parts, do not collapse nor are they convulsed but stay still, fixed, motionless and tense in the same position in which they were before attack. Gradually, or sometimes suddenly, normal motion returns. The senses and the normal animal activities are usually, but not always, diminished or abolished. This can be either with, or without, pain. It is accompanied by various spasmodic agitations in one part or another. I have observed such agitation in the nerves and muscles of the face, especially in the mouth and lips. The sick man wants to move his body sometimes but cannot. The disease is often accompanied by sadness of the mind.'

The immediate causes of this catalepsy are often anger, disgust, tedium, fright, terror and fear.

The relationship of catalepsy and depression was discussed by SCHOMBURG (Jena 1690). After a good review of literature he described the case of a 35-year-old woman who became depressed, fearful and anxious, then developed a stuporous episode, was mute, motionless and difficult to rouse. The author stressed the effect of terror which the patient had experienced at the beginning of the illness, emphasizing that women are prone to having terrifying phantasies. He related such experiences to ecstasy but emphasized that there is a difference between ecstasy and catalepsy.

In his dissertation, MANGOLDT (Basel 1673) wrote:

'In this affliction (catalepsy) the sick are taken ill suddenly and stiffen, devoid first of motion and then of sensation. They do not see although their eyes are fixed and open, and although they look like someone awake, the mind and the senses are in a stupor that they look as if they were suspended in admiration. Some people rather think that they are in some heaven than dead.'

As GLOCK emphasized:

'The absence of dreams, visions, not to mention other things show that our disorder (catalepsy) is not ecstasy.'

The clinical aspects and significance of ecstasy were reviewed fully by STOLTERFOHT (Greifswald 1692).

'They are not far wrong who take ecstasy to be a singular and violent commotion and alienation of mind in which the victims seem to be placed outside themselves, so that they lie for hours or days in a profound sleep. Although you may strike them, they are either not aroused or aroused with difficulty. The condition is accompanied by the symptoms described below.' ...

'I trust that no one will deny that there is a kind of diabolical ecstasy since, sadly, we see plenty of samples of demoniacs or people obsessed by the devil whom we see agitated by the devil in a thousand fashions. At one moment their mouths are twisted; at another we find the devil acting on the body itself and swelling it up.

'But leaving aside the things which do not ordinarily come under medical care, we beg pardon only of those who are in the habit of using terms precisely for having used the terms ecstasy and enthusiasm as synonyms in this dissertation although we are aware that theological meaning of the word enthusiasm is an unusual divine inspiration or occult sudden praeternatural knowledge of something infused by some spirit or demon.

'Hence, lest we wander aimlessly in tracking down one kind or another of similar disorders, we will describe exstasy or enthusiasm as a disorder in an extraordinary concentration of Archei[13], accompanied by temporary loss of sensation and motion, sometimes followed by certain visions. It originates from some unusual idea impressed on the imagination with a concomitant mental sympathy.'

'The ecstatic, although he lack sensation and motion, does not have accompanying spasms. He lies as if asleep with his eyes sometimes open but more often closed. However, we rarely observe convulsive motions but rather more natural ones.' ...

'It happens that they imagine things wholly incompatible and absurd, since their imagination actively proposes false images to them, or that they think and judge falsely. Hence, they have a diversity of concepts and fabricate many exotic ideas. Their mistakes may be grave as when, for example, they doubt their own existence (but not the way DESCARTES did). Sometimes they fancy an unusual meta-

13   VAN HELMONT postulated that each material process of the body is presided over by a special archaeus or spirit. PARACELSUS had given the term archeus to the vital principle.

morphosis; sometimes they idly glory in the receipt of royal honors; sometimes they are vexed by anxieties and sadness to the point where they even despair of salvation. It is not unusual for them to lay violent hands on themselves.'

STOLTERFOHT had difficulty in delineating the ecstatic picture and relates it to enthusiasm which he does not succeed in defining. He emphasized that in ecstasis and enthusiasm there is 'a loss and sometimes even an injury to sensation and motion' and assumes therefore that 'the whole nervous system is suffering'. Although these authors recognize that ecstasy may occur in mania, melancholia and epilepsy, inconsiderable clinical understanding was obtained until the second part of the 18th and early 19th centuries.

The treatment of catalepsy and ecstasy followed well-established lines and BOERHAAVE in his *Aphorism* (1709)[14] and VAN SWIETEN, in his elucidations, give as cause the immovability of the sensorium commune which continues to send forth its supply of spirits to these nerves that were in action at the time when the disease first invaded (aph. 1037). All function of the brain are disturbed, and dissections (aph. 1041) reveal that arteries and veins are turgid with thick blood forcibly driven into them. One should try to rouse the patient by objects which act powerfully upon the organ of the senses such as light, sound, a stimulus, acrid volatile salts, pain, friction, and continued motion. Hemorrhages from the nose should be promoted, as well as hemorrhoidal and menstrual discharges, sneezing powders to evacuate phlegm, medication to induce vomiting, blisters, issues, setons and moistening diet are recommended (aph. 1046). VAN SWIETEN also recommends wine and brandy and, if strong emotions are present, activity, diversion and travels.

In the 16th and 17th centuries venesectio in remote parts of the body (feet), stimulation of menstrual and hemorrhoidal flow, laxatives and resolvents were considered indicated, and attention to the correction of faulty natural and non-natural causes (see, e.g., KHONN, SCHOMBURG, BOLLMANN). There was no essential therapeutic change during this period.

14 BOERHAAVE, *op. cit.*

Chapter VI
Hysteria and Hypochondriasis

1. Hysteria

Hysteria as defined in the older literature deals with a group of symptoms which center around sensations in the abdomen and of suffocation in the chest. The patients complained of movement and often related pains in the abdomen, and of a ball which rested in the lower abdomen or moves upwards. The chest complaints referred to palpitation, pressure in the cardiac region, choking sensations and anxiety. The Greek and Roman authors explained the suffocation and the abdominal symptoms by a disorder of the uterus which caused it to rise and lead to fits of suffocation. Other symptoms, including pathological ones, were considered secondary. Although HIPPOCRATES and GALEN pointed out the protean changes in symptomatology, the uterine suffocation as well as its explanation by a uterine disorder were accepted as the leading principles until the 18th century.

The term hysteria, deriving from the Greek word for uterus, was used by HIPPOCRATES and GALEN. Later terms were suffocatio uterina or hysterica, strangulatio or strangulatus uteri, praefocatio (suffocation) uteri. Passio hysterica (hysterical suffering) was used in dissertations of the 18th century, indicating the change which had taken place when the disorder became related to the brain and nervous system. The adjective, hysterica was used either because the disorder was based on a uterine disturbance or because the author wanted to indicate that he discussed the same illness which previous authors, expecially HIPPOCRATES, had called hysteria.

The dissertations of the 16th, and those to the end of the 17th centuries referred to the textbook of RIVIÈRE[1] as the main source of reference. RIVIÈRE who followed the teachings of HIPPOCRATES and GALEN was greatly influenced by PLATTER and SENNERT. He wrote that 'the seed

1   RIVIÈRE, *op. cit.*

and menstrual blood may be retained in women' becoming putrefied and corrupted and venomous vapors arising from it. In addition, 'diverse humors of an excrementitious nature' may flow into the uterus and, when staying there a long time, putrefy and send out noxious vapors. This occurrence explains hysteria in older women in whom menstruation and production of seed has stopped. With amenorrhea in a young woman, noxious humors develop from corruption of the retained blood and seed. RIVIÈRE gives a detailed discussion of the symptoms, especially the attacks of feeling strangled which may occur with varying frequency and duration and are precipitated by sweet odors and the eating of meat and by anger, terror and emotional suffering. The choking may be caused by vapors compressing the lungs, by a combination of hysteria with hypochondriacal melancholia or by a special property of venomonous vapors. When they reach the brain and hinder the influx of animal spirits, the muscles serving respiration and the diaphragm are inhibited. He is critical of the statements of the older writers that the uterus can ascend, and offers a good differential diagnostic discussion of various symptoms, e.g., fainting, epilepsy and apoplexy.

During a fit of suffocation the patient should be put on a bed, with neck and shoulders elevated and the region of the sexual organs and the legs kept low.

The lower abdomen should be tied tightly, rubbed and chafed, and a cupping glass put to the hip. Strong and fetid odors, e.g., from burnt leather or asa foetida, are put to the nose or pepper put into the nose. One must, however, be careful not to use strong stimuli in a convulsion because they might stir up too much commotion in the brain. Laxatives and clysmas (enema) are to be used for removing the noxious vapors which cause the fits. RIVIÈRE warns against frequent blood letting in a weakened person. If retention of 'seed' is the cause, marriage is recommended (he disapproved of the accepted custom of tickling the cervix by a mid-wife). The use of wine is left in dispute, recommended by HIPPOCRATES, forbidden by AVICENNA. Cream of tartar and vitriolated steel (vitriolum Martis) is advised.

An early dissertation on hysteria was written by WOLFHARD (Basel 1604) who followed the Renaissance writers and GALEN, presenting as the cause the retention of the female 'semen' (due to lack of or infrequent intercourse) and menstrual blood. He distinguished between general symptoms which included the inactive senses, minimal convulsive movements and fainting, and special symptoms, i.e., those which are re-

lated to respiratory difficulties. A typical early dissertation was presented by GUGGER (Basel 1607) who in 83 brief statements revealed a good
book knowledge while JENCKE (Basel 1616) and GEISELBRUNNER (Basel
1622) offered a good discussion of the literature of the 16th century.

A group of dissertations from Leyden illustrate the current theories
and treatment and their critical non-dogmatic acceptance. VAN DER
MAST (Leyden 1650) presents briefly the case of a 30-year-old widow,
pointing out the differences from epilepsy and quoting GALEN's and FER-
NEL's opinions, who believed in the ascension of the uterus and RI-
VIÈRE's treatment. The dissertation of GESENIUS (Leyden 1654) uses as
illustration the case of a 28-year-old woman who in the bereavement of
her husband's death, had well described hysterical fits. The symptoms
are critically reviewed and their treatment, based on HIPPOCRATES and
GALEN, outlined in detail. SEELIGER (Leyden 1662) followed VAN HEL-
MONT's thinking and quoted SENNERT's discussion in his textbook. The
symptoms are caused by bad and dangerous vapors which originated
from bad humors in the uterus, corrupted by retained menstrual blood
and 'semen'. This well-organized dissertation presents the proximal and
remote and the natural and praeternatural causes. The description of
symptoms singles out the imminent signs and their development into the
sensations of strangulation. The carefully outlined treatment offers a
good understanding of the procedures and medications used at that time.

In this period a group of dissertations which distinguished between
hysterical and hypochondriacal suffocation was also accepted at Leyden.
They will be discussed later under the topic of hypochondriasis. The
medical faculty of Leyden was greatly interested in furthering the knowledge on hysteria and tried to maintain an unbiased attitude. Among
the leaders was the carefully observing clinician DE LE BOË (SYLVIUS),
whose student, WILLIS, brought about a great change in the theory and
clinical study of hysteria.

The publication by THOMAS WILLIS[2] of his *Pathologiae cerebri et
nervosi generis specimen* (1667) and of his answer to HIGHMORE's criticism (1670) greatly influenced the medical literature. In this connection
it is interesting to compare two dissertations from Erfurt, both written in
1672 under the praesidium of GEORG CHRISTOPH PETRI. The dissertation
of BERCKE (Erfurt 1672) was presented in March and that of GOTTER

2   WILLIS, *op. cit.* He attempted to correlate outstanding psychopathologic
symptoms with physiologic changes. In the treatment he stressed the need to correct the acidity by use of chemical drugs in addition to herbals.

(Erfurt 1672) in November. BERCKE still followed the teachings which had been presented in the publication of RIVIÈRE with a brief reference to SYLVIUS. GOTTER offered the views of WILLIS and discussed them concisely.

WILLIS included hysterical fits among the convulsive disorders because all of them were caused by the disordered animal spirits in the brain. This theory was attacked by HIGHMORE[3] who in 1660 had explained the hysterical suffocation as the rushing of blood into the lungs. The theory of WILLIS postulated that the animal spirits are in the center of the nerves and through their movements transmit sensory and motor impulses. He explained these spirits on a chemical basis. The opinion of most physicians of the previous centuries that the hysterical suffocation was caused by the upward movement of the uterus had, in literature, been questioned repeatedly on an anatomical basis, but never as emphatically as by WILLIS. Strong emotional experiences may disturb the spirits and make them receptive for noxious influences which may come from the uterus or other parts of the body. He accepted that retention of menses or female 'semen' or fluor albus may lead to stagnation of the fluid in the nerves and cause the disposition to a convulsive disorder (WILLIS' concept of convulsive disorder is broadly conceived, including epilepsy, hysteria, convulsive coughing, asthma and all convulsions in childhood). This formulation of hysteria was widely accepted because it was part of the development of neuro-anatomy as well as anatomy and pathology in general during the 17th century. The assumption that the center of the disturbance was in the brain had been mentioned by LE POIS (1563–1633) and SYDENHAM but not elaborated and no reference seems to have been made to them in students' dissertations although they quote these authors in other connections. SENNERT and others had stressed the immovability of the fixed uterus. As can be seen from dissertations in the 17th century the role of the uterus was questioned repeatedly when the symptoms were also described in men. In several dissertations the term suffocatio hypochondriaca was used as synonymous with hysteria, applied to men, and occasionally also to women.

In looking over the dissertations from 1670 to 1700 one notices two developments: a broader and more careful description of symptoms than previously, and an increasing attention to emotions. MORRIS (Leyden 1676) mentions the symptoms of lassitude of the whole body, yawning,

---

3   HIGHMORE, *op. cit.*

stretching, weakness of the legs, pale face, sad and fearful expression, a cold sensation which starts in the lumbar region and extends to the scapula, a cold feeling of the whole body and of the extremities, disturbances of internal and external senses and of mobility, headache, vertigo, tinnitus, anxiety and pressure in the heart region, palpitation, thin, weak and slow pulse, difficulty in breathing and often a sense of no breathing and marked fear of suffocation, constriction, strangulation of the throat, repugnance to food, nausea and vomiting, eructation of acid, bilious and rancid humors, rumbling in the abdomen, flatus, contortions and distensions in the abdomen, distension and pain in chest, abdomen and left hypochondrium. This enumeration of symptoms is quite in contrast to the brief description of hysterical fits in the older dissertations and in textbooks. The diversity of symptoms in hysteria has now become accepted. The differential diagnosis to epilepsy, apoplexy, catalepsy and fainting attacks becomes clearer and critical evaluation of the findings possible. The movements in the abdomen and tremors can be recognized as related to the bowels and not to the uterus. These discussions reveal a good knowledge of the literature on physiology and anatomy (SCHMID, Jena 1681). It became possible to distinguish these so-called tremors from tremors of the liver and illnesses of the hypochondrium.

The observation that emotional disturbances, especially fear, anxiety, worry and sadness precipitate attacks had been recognized by early writers on hysteria. In dissertations of the period under discussion the emotional symptoms of hysteria are emphasized, especially the emotional lability, the readiness to respond with crying and excessive laughter, unrestrained emotional display and vehement emotional behavior (LINCKE, Frankfurt a. O. 1678). These observations had been mentioned in the medical literature but now the students became aware of their significance and referred to them. BEHRENS (1684), e.g., quotes the observation of MONTANUS[4] that hysterical paroxysma occur due to fear, terror, sadness and at sudden death of friends. The dissertation of DE RHODA (Jena 1696) described in careful detail opisthotonus which had been mentioned by RIVIÈRE but was insufficiently described. This symptom corresponds to the 'horrible and inhuman convulsion' of other authors. Convulsions were considered caused by the influence of demons and treated accordingly, with the convictions and cruelty of the period, when the patient demonstrated contortions or gesticulations of the extremities

4 MONTANUS, op. cit.

or of the whole body which no healthy person could imitate (WAXMANN, Jena 1687).

After about 1700 most dissertations treated hysteria and hypochondriasis together. HAHN (Jena 1701) presented the case of a 28-year-old woman, who on the fifth day after childbirth complained of poor appetite and a feeling of strangulation and acute anxiety and began to have a trembling of her right arm and foot. Her voice was weak, her eyes staring and she was afraid of fainting. After a few days there was improvement of these symptoms but she now complained of periodic constrictions in the umbilical region, tremors in the lower abdomen and globus, and she looked terrified. The case is discussed on the basis of the writings of WILLIS and HIGHMORE. The author stressed that both, uterus and hypochondrium are involved and that hysterical symptoms are seen in male and female patients.

Another case, described by ZECH (Erfurt 1703) is that of a 40-year-old woman who complained of nausea, headache, vertigo, clouded vision, abdominal distension, rumbling in the abdomen, globus-like constrictions of the intestines and choking in her throat. She was in a state of debility. Her symptoms were relieved by induced vomiting and diarrhea, followed by fainting. She was restored to strength by a careful diet of wine and a small amount of bread. The author explains the clouded vision, vertigo and lassitude by the patient's sadness, anger and anxiety, and attributes the abdominal symptoms to her general physical condition which he calls scorbutic illness. The fainting was caused by the diarrhea and lack of sufficient food.

GERHARD (Groningen 1703), who distinguished hysteria in women from hypochondriasis in men discusses melancholic constitution as an important factor. In the usual list of symptoms he includes delirium, which one finds also mentioned in other dissertations of this period. These authors, however, do not define delirium and one can only assume that they observed some psychopathological symptoms but not whether the patients were briefly delirious or delusional. It is a fair statement that the psychopathological descriptions and understanding by the students rarely equalled that of the greatly admired SYDENHAM (1681)[5] who wrote that hysteria occurs more frequently in women than in men and after enumerating the usual somatic complaints and signs, mentions fits of laughter and crying. 'She shrieks irregularly, and inartic-

5   VEITH, op. cit., SYDENHAM, op. cit.

ulately, and strikes her breast' and 'has to be held down by the united efforts of the bystanders'. The patients feel dejected. 'Their mind sickens more than the body. An incurable despair is so thoroughly the nature of this disease, that the very slightest word of hope creates anger ... They have melancholy fore-bodings. They brood over trifles, cherishing them in their anxious and unquiet bosoms. Fear, anger, jealousy, suspicion, and the worst passions of the mind arise without cause ... there is no moderation. All is caprice. They love without measure those whom they soon will hate.'

It is interesting to note the increasing awareness of emotional insta-bility and the need to consider the emotions in the explanation of some of the symptoms and in the treatment. JARVIS (Edinburgh 1744) men-tions as important symptoms of sadness, insecurity, fluctuations in think-ing, lapses of memory, disturbed phantasies, suspicions of friends, feel-ing unjustly treated, sudden changes from tearfulness to excessive cheer-fulness. This is a considerable step forward from the enumeration of physical symptoms, with neglect of the psychological factors and reac-tions. Another striking feature of this period is the careful discussion of literature, especially of WILLIS and SYDENHAM but also a reference to DE LE BOË (SYLVIUS), LEPOIS (PISO) and RIVIÈRE. The case descriptions are usually longer than the observations in the publications of the learned societies and are a valuable contribution to literature.

The treatment follows the rules of the prominent physicians of the various periods leading among them GALEN, RIVIÈRE, DE LE BOË (SYL-VIUS), and WILLIS. In a thesis from Paris, CHAUVEL (Paris 1674) propos-es a therapeutic procedure which is still recommended in the medical lit-erature of the present century, the obtainment of much needed sexual satisfaction.

'The female uterus so hungrily craves the male seed that it is not to be won-dered that as a result of its absence hysterical symptoms are produced ... Suppres-sion of the menstrual blood is not to be thought of as the other cause of the hys-terical symptoms ... However frightful hysterical symptoms may be, their cure is still easy when the remedy of Venus is applied ... In hysterical women who are devoutly chaste the future is unhappy unless reason and honor suggest to them moments in which they can temper the fire of their burning uterus, but a cure like this pertains to the moral philosopher, not to the physician.'

In some dissertations medications which were especially recom-mended in the student's environment are discussed. An example is found in DELESTRE's (Montpellier 1711) recommendation of martialia of

Montpellier, an iron preparation which probably included some opium. There are many dissertations which in discussions of physical illnesses are devoted to justifying the therapeutic superiority of certain wines or beers, mineral waters or various medicaments. A perusal of past and current medical literature demonstrates that this type of publication is not limited to certain periods of medical history nor to dissertations.

2. Hypochondriasis

The term hypochondriacal affection relating to abdominal disorders was used by the Greek and Latin writers as well as by the Arabs, who called it affectus mirachialis. These abdominal complaints were found to be the outstanding symptoms in some depressions which were designated hypochondriacal melancholia. SENNERT seems to have been the first author who recognized that some patients have these complaints without depression being a dominant feature.

The terms, used at various times in literature are morbus hypochondriacus, affectio hypochondriacus, passio hypochondriaca and malum hypochondriacum. Passio hypochondriaca and malum hypochondriacum may refer to pains related to abdominal inflammation or to tumors while in some dissertations signify hypochondriasis. Under the influence of DE LE BOË (SYLVIUS) suffocatio hypochondriaca was assigned to men who had symptoms which corresponded to suffocatio hysterica in women.

In the Renaissance period hypochondriasis was recognized in connection with melancholia, i.e. depressions and schizophrenia. Several authors describe well the symptoms of what later was called hypochondriasis. The following description is taken from PLATTER's *Observationes*[6] (p. 33) under the title *Hypochondriac Melancholy, with Strange Imaginations:*

'These patients are convinced that they have various diseases, and some are true, others imaginary. This is especially true of men who are intelligent and delve into matters deeply, especially physicians that study the causes of diseases. They suppose they have these diseases, and tire out the physicians by telling about them, some write and talk that every part of their body, internally and externally, was diseased when, however, they can eat, sleep and drink well. They also may persuade themselves that they have lost all their natural heat and have many imaginary diseases in their brain, stomach, lungs, liver, kidneys. Some patients have

6   PLATTER, *op. cit.*

complained that they cannot sneeze, perspire or dream. Others complain of some true diseases but in addition they imagine many others. This is what I saw happen to a certain nobleman who for forty years tortured himself almost continuously with this kind of thoughts and used many remedies and who, nonetheless, lived to an advanced age.'

PLATTER's description fits well the later concept of hypochondriasis. One of his students, COLERUS (Basel 1608) in a discussion of scorbut and hypochondriacal flatulence describes the following symptoms: Nausea, vomiting of poorly digested food, sour and burning eructation, a feeling of tension (in the abdomen) and of heat, pressure on the chest with dyspnoea, orthopnoea and over-excitement, timidity, sadness, and terrible insomnia. He relates these symptoms more to the later concept of hypochondrias than hypochondriacal melancholia. One has to keep in mind that sadness (tristitia) meant all kinds and degrees of depressive feelings. Until the 19th century scorbut and hypochondriasis were related to each other. Many symptoms due to inanition were called scorbut.

BURCKHART (Basel 1630) offers a careful review of the literature and enumerates the symptoms which are found in hypochondriasis: Sour eructation, rumbling in the abdomen, flatulence, increased salivation, nausea, vomiting of sour and sticky phlegm, indigestion, voracious appetite, praecordial anxiety and palpitation, feeling of heat in the body, headache, diminished eyesight, often the feeling that the condition was getting worse, fear of impending apoplexy or death and continuously suffering from sad imagination. The treatment which he outlines follows PLATTER who recommended bleeding to stimulate menstruation and flow from the hemorrhoids, clysma, medicines to assuage the gastro-intestinal unrest and to induce vomiting. Sleep and activities should be moderated, and therapeutic sexual intercourse is recommended by some and condemned by others. Attention should be paid to disturbing emotions, especially irritability and sadness.

Under the influence of DE LE BOË (SYLVIUS) several dissertations from Leyden were devoted to hypochondriacal suffocation. VAN DYCK (Leyden 1665) mentioned as immediate causes acidity of vapors, breath and flatus, and as remote causes mucus, bile and pancreatic juice. Bile is affected by anger and mucous and the acid spirits by sadness and worrying. Other disturbing factors are cold air, unsatisfactory food and drink, sleep and rest and excretion. VERMEIREN (Leyden 1668) confirms his teacher's doctrines and outlines his therapeutic procedures. He stresses the importance to distinguish suffocation from syncope, apoplexy, epilepsy, incubus (fearful dreams with pressure of the chest) and from death. Other dissertations on this topic offer little in addition to what had been published, except additional references to literature of the 16th and 17th centuries. BLUM (Leipzig 1683), under the influence of ETTMÜLLER[7], followed SYLVIUS but stressed that the spleen becomes affected. He discusses the various kinds of pain of which the patient complains and how it can be explained and treated. The treatment is offered in a well-organized form.

The influence of HIGHMORE and WILLIS is already present in the dissertations of KORNMESSER (Rostock 1665), BLEKER (Kiel 1673), VOIGT (Prague 1675). The latter offers an unusually good discussion of literature of the 17th century as well as of the Greek, Latin and Arabic authors.

In the dissertations after 1670 the teaching of WILLIS[8] is fully accepted and the influence of SYDENHAM and BOERHAAVE becomes noticeable. The contributions from anatomical and pathological studies are stressed and clinical observations and their interpretations are critically made. MOHR (Rinteln 1678) evaluates abdominal pains in relationship to disturbed digestion and distension of the stomach, the influence of anxiety on the activities of the bowels, and the effect of troublesome emotions on sleep, dreams (incubus) and imagination. He mentions the frequency of seminal discharge. Hypochondriasis may result in melancholia hypochondriaca but rarely in mania. In the later dissertations various symptoms are stressed more or less. It may be that this selection was made for unimportant reasons but it is also possible that the patients' complaints changed because of still poorly understood factors. Such changes in symptomatology in psychoses and psychoneuroses have attracted little attention. Even when studies have been published, e.g., in connection with witchcraft, they have not been followed by further investigations from different points of view. In the dissertation of VAN BUREN (Leyden 1711) in addition to the gastro-intestinal complaints, pain in the dorsal and lumbar region are emphasized as well as headaches and vertigo. He mentioned the chronicity of the disorder. GRIFFITH (Leyden 1725) under the influence of SYDENHAM's teaching, reviews chronicity and intermittent courses and the effect of the many strong emotions which he quotes from the book of RIVIÈRE.

7   ETTMÜLLER, op. cit.
8   WILLIS, op. cit.

Toward the end of the 17th century hypochondriacal symptoms were found to occur frequently among scholars, and the term malum and morbus literatorum came into use. The explanation offered for this occurrence of suffocatio hypochondriaca was the sedentary life and the retention of the hemorrhoidal flow (stressed by BOERHAAVE and VAN SWIETEN)[9]. WALTERUS (Leyden 1688) discussed this aspect of hypochondriasis and ZIEGLER (Basel 1697) also referred to it when he discussed the case of a hard-working student who had little physical activity. He slackened in his work, felt depressed and complained of indigestion, of a bitter taste in his mouth, occasional vomiting of mucus, eructation, abdominal pain, constipation and palpitation. This illness was distinguished from the ill-defined scorbut, melancholia hypochondriaca and passio hysterica. The illness of the scholars became increasingly recognized in German medicine of the 18th and 19th century. The dissertation of HEYMAN (Leyden 1732) emphasized the patient's attention to health – with its attendant apprehension and anxiety, fixed preoccupations and avoidance of even minor physical exertion. Dissertations and later discussion in book form occasionally include what would now be considered catatonic and schizophrenic illnesses as well as mild depression.

Starting toward the end of the 17th century in medical books and dissertations emphasis was put on attention to minor discomforts, especially of the gastro-intestinal tract, and the regimen of diet. (This term compares well with the current psychiatric concept of a healthy routine of living, with its stress on a balance of psychological and physical factors.) In the second part of the 18th century the books of TISSOT and ACKERMANN[10] exerted a wide influence on the medical and educated lay groups.

In the 18th century hypochondriasis and hysteria were no longer considered essentially different and no sharp differentiation between the symptoms was maintained. The dissertations of STOCHIUS (Utrecht 1730), BOBIN (1745) and STOCKMANN (Halle 1747) well illustrate this development. Malum hypochondriacum is now the chronic illness of men in which the blood flow in the visceral blood vessel is impeded,

---

9   BOERHAAVE, op. cit.
10   TISSOT, S. A., Advice to the people in general with regard to their health, Dublin 1766; De la santé des gens de lettres, Lausanne 1769.
ACKERMANN, JOHANN CHRISTIAN GOTTLIEB, Über die Krankheiten der Gelehrten, Nürnberg 1777.

malum hystericum the chronic illness of women with impeded abdominal blood flow. Under STAHL's influence[11] the psychopathological symptoms were increasingly related to emotions.

3. Somnambulism

Walking in the sleep is a phenomenon which has puzzled physicians since the Greek and Latin period. One finds such occurrences described in the observations of the 16th and 17th centuries which were frequently quoted in the dissertations of this topic. AB HEER (1631)[12] mentions the case of a young poet. One night, after having been frustrated in expressing himself in verse to his satisfaction, he went to sleep. While asleep he got up, walked to his desk and wrote happily the lines which he had not been able to do previously. The next morning he had amnesia for this episode. A few years later his wife observed that, with his eyes open but apparently asleep, he went to take his infant son from the crib. Somnambulism recurred until the age of 45 when it stopped completely. JACOB HORST (1593)[13] discussed somnambulism in a treatise which attracted much attention. He describes a man who in his sleep walked downstairs, crossed a large courtyard and stepped into the fountain. He held himself strongly with his hands on the wall of the fountain and walked securely (on the wet stones). He did not enter the water but the hem of his shirt became wet and the cold water probably woke him up. HORST also mentions a young man who, wandering in his sleep, broke his leg.

PLATTER[14] discussed the state between sleeping and awake in which complicated and well-coordinated activities can be carried out and cannot be remembered. (This observation was confirmed and emphasized by RIBOT – 1885.)

SENNERT[15] reviews somnambulia, basing his discussion on JACOB HORST's treatise but also including other authors, among them PROSPER ALPINUS[16]. In many textbooks cases of somnambulism were mentioned

11 STAHL's influence is discussed in chapter IX, psychopathology.
12 AB HEER, *op. cit.*
13 HORST, *op. cit.*
14 PLATTER, *op. cit.* Praxeos. This observation was confirmed and emphasized by TH. RIBOT, *Les maladies de la mémoire,* Paris 1885.
15 SENNERT, *op. cit.* lib. II, part III, sect. II, cap. IV.
16 PROSPER AEGINUS, *De medicina Aegyptorum,* Venice 1591.

but without offering additional observations. It was stressed that a person in a somnambulistic state can achieve dangerous feats which he could not perform while awake, e.g. walking a narrow ledge high above the ground. Some patients are able to walk for a considerable period of time and carry out involved tasks. Much weight was placed on the fact as to whether the eyes were wide open or nearly closed. Usually the patient acts alone but there are references in literature to the fact that sometimes children and adolescents may walk in their sleep with one or more companions who sleep in the same room. WEPFER (1650)[17] mentions two nuns who, in their sleep but with their eyes open, walked together through the monastery, up and down stairs and lighted candles. Like all cases of somnambulism these two nuns had complete amnesia for their acts.

The first dissertation which I found in literature was by GEORG HORST (Wittenberg 1602) who discussed sleep walking with interesting references in literature. He mentioned the effect of imagination in the voluntary muscles and the temperature of the humors. Thus, he tried to explain the effect of strong emotions and desires in dreams on activities stimulated and carried out while asleep. The causes might be divine or natural, the latter including the effect of seeds of papaver and of alcohol. The role which alcoholic intoxication might play in sleep walking had already been mentioned by the Renaissance physician, FRACASTORIUS[18]. GEORG HORST made an attempt to correlate the symptoms of somnambulism with the available knowledge of brain anatomy.

Several dissertations were written during the 17th century. HOFSTETTER (Halle 1695) emphasized that the spirits are the chain between body and soul (anima). He presented in detail the cases of JACOB HORST and AB HEER and added his own observation of a 12-year-old boy who had taken much alcoholic beverage the preceding evening. In his sleep he walked through an open window and was killed. In the opinion of the author these patients seem deliberately to act not by mental judgment but purely by imagination and the ruling of the senses. He discussed in detail the literature of the 18th century, including brief case descriptions found in the *Miscellanea Curiosa* of the Academia Caesarea-Leopoldina. In this dissertation which was written under the direction of FRIEDRICH HOFFMANN, the author postulates that somnambulism is a state between being fully awake and asleep. At the same time and in

17   WEPFER, *op. cit.,* obs. XVIV.
18   HIERONYMUS FRACASTONIUS, *Opera omnia*, Venice 1584.

the same university STAHL theorized that the disorder was caused by the accumulation of too much blood in the vessels of the brain, which slowed the blood flow and resulted in obstructions, leading to corruptions of the phantasy. He spoke of noctambulatio naturalis when the patient carried out activities of his daily life, and of noctambulatio praeternaturalis when unusual activities or unusual places were involved. By several authors the influence of the moon on somnambulism had been mentioned in literature and this theory was strongly supported by MEAD (1702). In his dissertation WIPPACHER (Leipzig 1717) accepted this usually rejected theory when he reviewed the case of a medical student. At night as well as in the daytime as soon as he fell asleep sitting in his chair, he stood up, turned pages in his notebook, took Castelli's Lexicon and looked for the explanation of medical terms. He cursed when he could not find them. Otherwise he copied them happily and when he had finished sat down again asleep. This type of patient with his complicated purposeful activities and dramatic display of emotions invited discussions as to whether one dealt with stimulation or with unconscious activities. The development of hypnosis towards the latter part of the century confronted the physicians with the induced state of somnambulism and the same type of dispute was continued. Again with the increasing acceptance of the clinical picture of hysteria in the 19th century the discussion of the meaning of somnambulism was renewed.

A detailed review of the literature with the inclusion of various case presentations by authors of the preceding centuries was offered by STEPHANI (Basel 1701); it is always interesting to note how little the medical treatment in psychiatric conditions has changed during the 17th and early 18th century. In hysteria and hypochondriasis as well as in somnambulism the therapeutic procedures, whatever the theoretical considerations, as outlined on page 3 persisted. The increasing interest in the use of baths is treated in the dissertation of THOME (Avignon 1713).

The possible danger to others by an attack from a somnambulistic patient is a recurrent topic in literature. The case of SCHOTT[19] is often mentioned: A school teacher who in his sleep repeatedly talked loudly to his students, admonishing and scolding them. His roommate threatened to whip him if he continued to disturb his sleep. The following night the teacher got up, took a large pair of scissors, went to the other man's bed and stuck the scissors several times into the pillow. He then returned to

19   SCHOTT, CASPAR, *Physica curiosa*, Würzburg 1667.

his bed to sleep. Fortunately the roommate had been awake and was able to slip out of the bed. The patient said the next morning that he had dreamed that his roommate had tried to whip him and he had taken the scissors to defend himself. He had complete amnesia for the actual occurrence. In dissertations of the second half of the 18th century when legal medicine was finding a place in German medical schools several dissertations dealt with the topic of attacks on others and whether the patient was not responsible for his acts as ZACCHIAS (1584–1659)[20] had postulated or whether one dealt with simulation.

20 ZACCHIAS, *op. cit.*

Chapter VII
Psychopathological Disorders with Brain Tissue Damage

The psychiatric disorders which are grouped together in this chapter have in the history of medicine always been separated from the previously discussed illnesses. The pathological damage was definitely related to direct or indirect damage of the brain tissue. The point of direct and indirect brain damage becomes clarified in a discussion of delirium which comprises the two disorders, phrenitis and paraphrenitis.

1. Phrenitis and Paraphrenitis

In the 16th and 17th centuries delirium was defined as an illness which is characterized by depraved imagination and reasoning and judgment, i.e., expressed in hallucinations, delusions and poor judgement, These symptoms may occur in a variety of psychiatric disorders, including phrenitis, lethargy, melancholia, mania and stupiditas. There is, however, an important point which was stressed, the presence or absence of fever. If fever was present the symptoms were to be attributed to an inflammation of the brain and meninges. Its absence was necessary for the diagnosis of melancholia, mania or stupiditas. This last clinical entity began to lose importance in the 17th century. Lethargy was also unimportant psychiatrically because this syndrome was usually recognized as neurological.

Phrenitis was called delirium by Latin writers and both terms were later used interchangeably. Paraphrenitis referred to a delirium which had its origin located outside the cranial cavity.

A review of leading textbooks is important because teachers and students might use the terms differently according to the authority quoted. FERNEL[1] defined phrenitis as an inflammation of the meninges or of

---

1   FERNEL, *op. cit.*

the brain, causing fever and mental disorders. In a delirium these symptoms were caused by an illness outside the brain. PLATTER[2], in 1604, offered the following clarification:

'Phrenitis is delirium in which, just as in mania, the mind is quite alienated, but to a greater or lesser degree, depending on the gravity of the disorder. The victims reveal this alike in word and deed, for the moment they turn angry and rage with curses, cries and blaphemies and, like maniacs, long to injure someone. In these cases there is a peculiar phenomenon: they think, on account of a false imagination, that flies, bits of wool and straws are moving in front of their eyes and that various spectres are appearing to them, and they try to chase after them, catch at them, gather them, and cast them away.

But in addition to the disorders of this kind of a mind, which disorders are common also in mania, there come along with it other serious warm diseases, especially fever, which, if delirium (delirium) is added to it during the first attack, is called the disorder of phrenitis. But if that happens after the fever has already lasted for a while and headache has preceded, especially if it is continuous around the crisis, or if it first comes in the beginning or peak of the paroxysm and is intermittent, then it is called paraphrenitis.

Hence, along with delirium, which, as was said, is now very grave and now mild, continual fever symptoms also occur, more severe or more mild, as the heat of the fever becomes greater or milder, for example, on account of the heat of the heart: fast pulse, quick respiration, and fainting sometimes with sighs drawn at long intervals, on account of the inflammation of the natural parts: thirst and dryness of the tongue. But primarily, the causes of an overheated brain, apart from delirium, are insomnia, wakefulness, blurred vision and vertigo. If the brain is severely inflamed, as is mentioned under Causes, these become more severe and numerous.'

On page 13 the author refers briefly to sopor with delirium, stating that it is a condition in which the patient is awake and 'observes images

2   PLATTER, *op. cit.* Praxeos, cap. III. PLATTER seemed to follow GALEN who differentiated fever delirium from phrenitis, in which the brain is primarily affected, with a gradual development of psychopathological symptoms and not necessarily decreasing simultaneously with the subsiding of the fever. In fever delirium caused by a condition outside the brain one deals with a sudden onset of psychopathological symptoms and fever, both subsiding spontaneously if the brain has not become affected. GUAINERIO's predelirium which has its causes outside the brain, and is therefore called by him paraphrenitis, might be the early stage of a fever or toxic delirium. Both may prepare the way for a true delirium; i.e., inflammation of the brain or its membranes. In the succeeding centuries the term delirium was frequently applied to both phrenitis and paraphrenitis. The term predelirium does not seem to have been used, but in later dissertations it became accepted clinically that early psychopathological changes which may or may not lead to a full delirium must be recognized and treated.

and spectres of various things'. If they go to sleep they are troubled by terrifying dreams which they are able to relate when awake. Other terms for this condition are cataphora, coma agripnon and typhomania. PLAT-TER differentiates sopor with delirium from catatonia and ecstasy. In modern psychiatry sopor and delirium are discussed thoroughly but little study has been directed at a better psychodynamic and psychopathological understanding.

RIVIÈRE (1640)[3] defined phrenitis as an inflammation of the brain and its membranes, with a continuous mental derangement and fever. The brain might be directly affected by the sun (sunstroke), apoplexy, contusion, wine, anger. A secondary phrenzy might follow malignant fevers. He distinguished phrenitis from paraphrenitis in which hot distemper is communicated to the brain either from the whole body or from a part (i.e., from the stomach, liver, lungs, diaphragm).

Treatment essentially did not change during the period under discussion. RIVIÈRE recommended bleeding from the veins of the head or, if the hemorrhoids have stopped, from the foot. He advised limited but repeated bleeding while SENNERT urged large amounts of blood to be withdrawn at once. RIVIÈRE further used clysters and purging but only in secondary phrenitis. Repelling medicines were supposed to hinder the ascent of the humors and cool the head (among these medicines are oil of roses, violets or water lilies). He advised against giving cooling medicine which might make the naturally cool brain too cool and lead to coma. Instead, he prefered to cool the whole body by the use of juleps and emulsions, by washing the body and by footbath. Other authors deviated little from these recommendations which were followed by the students.

The earliest printed dissertations on phrenitis appeared before the textbooks of RIVIÈRE and PLATTER. At the University of Leipzig the internist, VON DREMBACH, put a question to GERITS (1571) with regard to the treatment of phrenitis. Referring to GALEN and HIPPOCRATES the student reviewed well, although in a condensed form, the concept and clinical picture and then explained clearly the treatment which in no essential way differed from the one found in the textbook of the early 17th century. In a dissertation from Basel where PLATTER and BAUHIN were already teaching the importance of careful anatomical and clinical observation, BRUNNER (Basel 1576) postulated that there were three types of

3   RIVIÈRE, *op. cit.*, lib. I (Praxeos med.), cap. XI.

phrenitis; the first was expressed by damage of the imagination which was related to lesions of the anterior part of the brain; the second by damage of reasoning and related to the midbrain, and the third by memory and related to the posterior part. He tried to explain symptoms on a physical basis, e.g., fearful hallucinations of beasts caused by black humors and more complicated symptoms by mixed humors. DIDYMUS (Basel 1583) attempted to differentiate clinically between phrenitis and paraphrenitis, considering the more marked degree of intensity of the symptoms characteristic of phrenitis. These considerations led to an emphasis on the early symptoms of phrenitis (marked insomnia, headache, and troublesome dreams, the content of which was not remembered) and of the full-fledged picture with visual hallucinations (grasping at light and straws) and increased fever and respiration. SCHROEDER (Kiel 1584) reviews the psychopathological symptoms more carefully and concludes that the main damage is of the imagination while the changes observed in reasoning and memory are less significant although many times very disturbing. GLASBERG (Basel 1591) contributed further to differential diagnosis, separating phrenitis exquisita from non-exquisita, the former caused by inflammation of the brain and meninges, the latter by hot vapors affecting brain and meninges. When yellow bile is present the delirium becomes more intense, leading even to mania (a marked excitement) and death. He evaluated the different symptoms in delirium, lethargy and mania. His interest, however, was more directed to a clearer formulation of pathogenesis than of the description of symptoms and treatment. BAUSCH (Basel 1601) tried to clarify the definitions of paraphrenia, mania and melancholia and presented a detailed review of treatment. In this period PLATTER worked on his textbook and the first part of it, dealing with the disturbances of senses and mobility (De functionum laesionibus, librio duos) appeared in 1602 and was reprinted without change in the *Praxeos medicae*. The psychiatric disorders are discussed in this part of the book. The passage on delirium quoted (see p. 2) may serve for comparison with dissertations which appeared when he was professor of medicine (1560–1619). It is surprising that his outstanding *Observationes* contain no example of delirium with the exception of a post-partum psychosis which he calls delirium but without offering convincing data to support this diagnosis. Among the causes PLATTER discussed toxic factors, including wine, beer and distilled wine, narcotics (hyoscyamus, mandragora, opium) and poisons, e.g., rabies. His next group included fever, especially if combined with pus, and inflammations of the body related to infectious diseases, and of the brain and meninges.

KRAPFF (Basel 1607) defined phrenitis as 'corrupted function of the main part of the brain'. Affected may be the anterior or middle part of the brain or both, and the symptoms are, therefore, depraved functions of the imagination or of reason, or both. (The author gives recognition to his three teachers PLATTER, STUPANUS and BAUHIN, the latter two known for their contribution in anatomy.) For the discussion of causes he followed PLATTER. In a dissertation by GILLENIUS (Basel 1609) the influence of GALEN and HIPPOCRATES is marked and few observations by the author are apparent. Following GALEN he mentions a type characterized by wrong thinking and judgment, another with sensory disorders and nearly intact thinking, and a third in which imagination and thinking are disturbed. HEINIUS (Basel 1609) gives a good discussion of the theories of GALEN and FERNEL and a good summary of the symptoms which are clearer and more discriminating than in PLATTER's book. After a beginning of disturbed sleep and dreams follows a clinical picture with overtalkativeness and silence, inattention and forgetting what had been said or done, fearfulness and at some times impudence (unusual behavior for this patient), answering irrationally to questions, exposing himself, gesticulating, pulling at straws or picking flakes of dust from his clothes, chasing flies and insects which the patient imagined in front of him. His expression was often wild and frightening. In this dissertation fear is stressed as an important emotion. SCHMITNER (Basel 1612) made an effort to distinguish between delusions as a part of a fever delirium and, without fever, in melancholia. Two dissertations which appeared after PLATTER's death, but while his influence in Basel was still great, offer a good review of pertinent literature, JUNCKER (Basel 1618), of the writers of the Latin and Arabian period and the early 16th century and FABRICIUS (Basel 1620) of the 16th century and early 17th century. While JUNCKER emphasized varying psychopathology in delirium, dependent on the strength or weakness of the brain for various causes, HUTTEN (Basel 1619) emphasized the variations which occur during the course of a delirium and the progression in severity until ending in death. (Both dissertations were written under BAUHIN as praeceptor.)

This group of dissertations from Basel offers a vivid picture of the increasing knowledge in the clinical psychopathology of delirium and of the carefulness with which various aspects were selected and treated. The period between 1620 and 1670 seems to have offered less new clinical knowledge[4]. AYRER (Jena 1632) confirmed the observations of HEINIUS and HUTTEN. VAN DER BUSCH (Leyden 1668) discussed three degrees of intensity of delirium: first, disturbance of vision (blurring); second, of thinking and perception; third, of judgment and memory. He further considered the emotional and intellectural disorders accompanying them, and confirmed that phrenitis is a continuous delirium with continuous fever which originates from inflammation of the meninges. Paraphrenitis is caused by fever from the inflammation of the diaphragm. He then discussed at length the differential diagnosis of mania, melancholia, lycanthropia, and somnambulism and the treatment of all these disorders. DOSE (Leyden 1671) gave much space to treatment as it had been outlined by RIVIÈRE. Following his teacher DE LE BOË, LOVELL (Leyden 1673) stressed the importance of bile, pancreatic juice and intestinal mucus and their corruption.

The interest in delirium became stimulated in the second half of the 17th century by the theoretical formulations of WILLIS, by findings in post-mortem investigations and the development of physiology. The result can be seen in the increased number of dissertations which dealt with delirium.

In a lengthy discussion WILLIS[5] defines phrenitis as a disorder arising from inflammation of the brain; i.e., of the animal spirits, and paraphrenitis as a disturbance of the animal and vital spirits in the (whole) brain which deprave and pervert every animal function.

'At the same time very many ideas of things being raised up out of the memory; the old are confounded with the new, and some evilly joined or wonderfully divided are confounded with others. The imagination suggests manifold phanthasms, and almost innumerable and all of them only incongruous.'

This description stimulated interest in the psychopathology of delirium which term is used now in literature, combining both phrenitis and paraphrenitis. He also emphasized that a delirium usually terminates in a short time in recovery or death. It may continue after the fever has ceased and pass into lethargy, mania or melancholia. The observations in medical literature and in his own experience led him to conclude that the causes are either too much heat or 'noxious matter' in the blood – fever, toxins (alcohol, mandrake, smallpox and plague) or insufficient animal spirits (after excessive hemorrhages, lack of sleep or food). WIL-

4   SENNERT, op. cit., lib. II, pact III, sect. II, cap. IV.
5   WILLIS, op. cit. (Transl. S. PORDAGE, The Soul of Brutes, p. 182).

LIS mentions in addition a 'hysterical delirium' which corresponds to the modern psychogenic delirium and which he characterized by the symptoms of swelling of the abdomen, oppression of the heart, talking idly with weeping and laughing. He postulated that disturbed animal spirits rise from the abdomen to the brain.

ESMARCH (Kiel 1681) and BENIER (Leyden 1682) reviewed the problem of phrenitis and paraphrenitis from the point of view of the theories of WILLIS. ESMARCH's teacher, PECHLIN was an excellent clinical observer with interest in psychopathology. It is therefore not surprising that this student carefully notes the psychopathological symptoms which he then tried to explain based on the theories of DESCARTES and WILLIS. He is one of the few writers who tried to understand hallucinations of fire, robbers and ghosts which were frightening or might be persons whom the patient hated or loved. The patient might watch them with astonishment as a novelty, with fear as if it were a danger, or as something absurd. Deliria differed in degrees of intensity, in the type of fever and in its course. Several other dissertations from followers of WILLIS offer little that was new but it is striking how often wine (probably brandy) and poisonous herbs were mentioned among the causes. The role of vehement emotions, especially anger, was also stressed. External injuries, e.g., concussions and marked loss of blood could lead to a disturbance of the spirits. Whatever could irritate the bile, corrupt or augment it, could produce a delirium. Depravation of phantasy is caused by depressed or exalted spirits. Supporting these statements CUMMIUS (Jena 1686) then formulated that depravation exists when pictures and objects which cannot be recognized by others are seen by the patient.

Dissertations of the 18th century, ZWINGER (Basel 1731), LINPRUNER (Göttingen 1747), OSCHWALD (Göttingen 1747), were essentially physiological with little reference to psychopathology. They are mentioned because they offer an understanding of the new theoretical concepts and their effect on clinical practice. Others, like PECK (Halle 1739) tried unsuccessfully to gain a better understanding from post-mortem studies. Phrenitis occurring in epidemics was no longer explained by changes in the air but related to unknown factors, present in certain regions. The possibility of toxic weeds was considered. It is interesting to note that these authors also considered the effect of phrenitis on an existing mania (excitement) and melancholia (including depression and schizophrenia). Transient changes in psychopathology were observed but could not yet be clearly enough described to permit an evaluation.

Treatment, as outlined by RIVIÈRE and by WILLIS was recommended in the dissertations, sometimes in detail, sometimes in a condensed form. None of the dissertations read made a contribution to therapy.

2. Disorders of Memory

In the medical literature since HIPPOCRATES memory has been discussed from the point of view of psychology and psychopathology. The brief summary offered by RIVIÈRE[6] may serve as an orientation:

'Memory is that operation of the soul which retains and preserves the received species of things. Reminiscence summons up those things that have left the memory, rallying them by the help of those which are yet retained.'

He stressed that memory is not merely a passive receptacle but consists of functions which are in progressive motion.

The terminology used includes memoria laesa (damaged memory), memoriae debilitas (weakness), memoriae deperditio (loss) and oblivio (forgetfulness) as well as terms referring to preservation of memory and damage to it.

In textbooks memory always received some discussion and observations by various authors quoted. They are usually brief but valuable because they include examples of head injuries, the effect of epilepsy and of toxic conditions, among them excessive alcoholism. The importance of heredity and congenital brain injuries was stressed.

During the ruling of humoral pathology the damage was explained by a cold distemper of the brain and excessive moisture of dryness. Other causes mentioned included excessive loss of blood, dietary mistakes, too much sleep, vomiting, diarrhea, intellectual idleness or excessive studying, worry and distraction by too many objects. The theoretical changes offered by WILLIS had little effect on the study and treatment of disorders of memory. In the Renaissance period strengthening the memory received much attention and mnemotechnical procedures and a healthy regime of living were recommended. As this advice also stressed the importance of correcting any, even minor, physical ailments and to restrict alcohol intake in old persons, the results may often have been noticed in better functioning of memory, attention and concentration.

6   RIVIÈRE, op. cit.

GIGAS (Basel 1602) offers a good review of the knowledge at that time. Separating congenital from acquired damage to memory he distinguishes three groups: abolished memory (amnesia for a period), obtuse and infirm memory, and depraved memory. The latter is discussed well, stating, e.g., that delirium may lead to memory lesion because there is insufficient proper retention because of the disturbed imagination and judgment. Forgetfulness occurs if the patient does not retain what he has perceived. Two dissertations were written simultaneously by CRUSCHIUS (Wittenberg 1609) and AEMYLIUS. The first dissertation discussed the preservation of memory. The Arabic physicians recommended conserving memory in beginning senescence by prescribing the blossoms and leaves of borage in wine or beer. The author prefered a 'rational protection', i.e. based on humoral pathology instead of the Arabic empiricism. The brain should be kept warm and free from excessive humidity or dryness by keeping a sound balance of sleep and being awake, moderate exercise and a healthy diet, including moderate consumption of alcohol. AEMYLIUS (Wittenberg 1609) mentioned as signs of a damaged memory that the patient has forgotten what he has previously known well and is astonished by hearing a discourse from literature with which he has been well acquainted, but which he does not remember. Other patients may only forget parts of what should be remembered. The treatment suggested included the prescription of the Arabic physicians, and the outlook for help was pessimistic.

No dissertations seem to have been presented until a strong interest developed with the progress of brain anatomy during the second part of the 17th century. MEIER (Basel 1687) carefully reviewed pertinent literature and applied the increasing knowledge of brain anatomy and clinical medicine to a re-evaluation of the concept of memory and forgetting. He stressed that emotional factors influence forgetting. His inaugural dissertation is called a meditation (meditatio) and quite correctly so. About half of his presentation is given to a detailed discussion of the use of medicines which were said to be helpful to strengthen memory.

BUDAEUS (Wittenberg 1686) after a discussion of the sensorium commune and the sensory basis of imagination and memory postulates a rational and sensual memory. The sensual memory deals with conservation, cognition and recall. Damage may be to the brain and to the substance of the spirits. Diminution of the memory is caused by difficulty in reception or by a loss of what has been received. Abolishment is due to inability of reception or of retention. The lesion may be in the brain or in interference with its functions. The latter occurs in cachexia, melancholia, and scorbut. Diminution may be caused by daily headaches, hydrocephalus, paralysis, epilepsy, apoplexy and fever, by poisons, by grave concussions, brain damage and old age. Hereditary factors should be considered, according to WILLIS. The impure air in certain countries (e.g. the Tyrol), dietary mistakes and intense terror and fear might be other causes. KAULIZIUS (Jena 1690) stressed the emotions and their effect on memory in sadness, excitements, melancholia and catalepsy. Treatment, outlined at length, must try to restore and free the spirits and then to preserve the viscid and acid humors. WOLFF (Jena 1696) reviewed the current knowledge of psychology and pathology of memory, and treatment at length. MALET (Jena 1696) is the only author who presented the history of a patient (the others referred to literature). A 20-year-old man, of cold and humid temperament, was born at a very unfortunate constellation of the stars. He consumed a great deal of alcoholic drinks, kept a bad diet, indulged in much sleep and sexual excesses. After a fall from a height he became aware of a decreased ability to remember what he had studied. When he had learned something he forgot it readily. His senses became slow; he lost his ambition. The discussion of this case summarized the essential symptoms, relating the memory defect to the injury of the occipital part of the brain. The immediate cause is the poverty and poor disposition of the spirits. Phlegm collected in the brain, causing somnolence. Among the remote causes he included the patient's cold and humid temperament and the astrological praedestination. His drunkenness and his sexual excesses contributed to the poor memory. The rapid forgetting of what he had read was related to insufficiency of the brain.

GILGIUS (Altdorf 1691) postulated that

'injury to the memory arising from too much sexual activity is a difficult and less prompt recall of the species previously represented in the common sensorium. It comes from a deficiency of the spirits which carry the species to the seat of the memory'.

He states that it is safe to conclude that memory is defective from excessive sexual activities if the patient had a good memory before he married and if after marriage his sexual indulgence was excessive.

Reviewing the dissertations on disturbance of memory one can see a group at the beginning of the 18th century in which the authors made an effort to clarify the sparse clinical data available. In the second group, at the end of the century, an effort was made to find a reformulation based on newly gained knowledge of the anatomy of the brain. There was also increased interest in a secondary type of disordered memory which was observed in phrenitis, mania and melancholia.

3. Psychopathology in Epilepsy

In medical literature there are frequent brief references that memory disorders may accompany epilepsy. FERNEL (consilia, 8)[7] mentions an 8-year-old boy who suffered for a long duration from epilepsy and whose intelligence and memory were affected by it. The relationship of such intense emotions as fear, anger and especially sudden fright was noticed frequently and also reported in the observations of many authors. A few authors mentioned a relationship of epilepsy with depressive reactions. The occurrence of convulsions at different phases of the moon was stressed, leading to considerable discussion in literature, and still strongly confirmed by MEAD in the 18th century.

Psychotic episodes, or lasting psychotic changes in epilepsy, were described by RULAND (1580)[8] who wrote that twice a year a patient had attacks in which, after an epileptic convulsion, he remained lying on the ground. Regaining his strength

'he fled through the forests, fields and other places in a state of madness, running this way and that, until his reason was restored and he returned home'. (Quoted by TEMKIN)[9].

This description is not very satisfactory. Descriptions with discussion of epileptic psychoses and psychopathology have apparently not appeared in literature before the second part of the 18th and especially in the 19th centuries. The dissertation of TILEMAN (Leyden 1677) contains a case description.

In the bibliography a few dissertations are mentioned. Epilepsia hysterica is an epilepsy of uterine origin. HEDENUS (Jena 1676) made this diagnosis because the epileptic convulsions were preceded by movements of the uterus and 'abdominal convulsions', anxiety which was referred to the cardiac region, difficulty in respiration and swallowing, a feeling of sadness and nightmares. Similar cases have been quoted re-

7 FERNEL, op. cit.
8 RULAND, op. cit.
9 TEMKIN, op. cit.

peatedly in literature, even in the present century and lead to lengthy discussions of the psychodynamics in epilepsy and hysteria. The question remained unanswered as to whether hysterical epilepsy was the development of epilepsy in a hysteria of several years duration as already Rivière had concluded in a woman described in his observations (centuria II, case 31)[10] or whether convulsions which were related to psychodynamic or somatic factors had occurred. Psychopathological symptoms and considerations are mentioned in epilepsia hypochondriaca and in epilepsy in relationship to melancholia.

4. Alcoholism

The recognition of alcoholism as a medical-social problem was increasingly discussed in medical and popular literature of the 16th and 17th centuries. In the preceding centuries alcoholism as an individual problem, especially acute intoxication, received attention. The authors of many textbooks discussed how one might prevent acute intoxication, and especially hangovers, suggesting vinegar and various herbs.

The publication of Schrick's (1481)[11] book, printed in German, outlined a simple process of distillation so that a housewife could make cheap brandy. The book was reprinted as late as 1530. Schrick, professor of medicine in Vienna recommended brandy in the amount of a half a (soup) spoon every morning – to stay in good health, to strengthen memory, reasoning and intelligence. Brandy was to be used for diseases of heart, liver, lungs, and bladder stones. His recommendations were widely followed by the 16th century physicians and by the people of Germany. The influential books of Conrad Gessner and Hieronymus Brunschwig reprinted them, adding that brandy was indicated for treatment of melancholia and mania. Another important factor of increasing alcoholism was the popularity of beer when the previously not very tasty drink was improved by the addition of hop. Beer and brandy became the alcoholic beverage in European countries where wine was not very good. In the wine-drinking countries of southern France and Italy alcoholism was less important than in northern Europe. The chronicles of

---

10   Rivière, op. cit.
11   Michael Schrick, Nützlich Büchlein von Kunst und Tugend der gebrannten Wasser, Nürnberg 1481.

that period described vividly the wide-spread drunkeness in Germany, the excesses in autumn festivals in the cities and towns, at the Kermess in the Low countries and the 'church-ales' in England. Alcoholism in women increased rapidly and children were permitted, or even advised to drink. Brandy was a cheap drink which replaced beer during hard economic times. During periods of famine, when wars and pestilence had damaged a country severely, the valuable grain food was used to make brandy. At the universities drinking was excessive among teachers and students and was attacked ineffectually by the academic leaders.

In 1516 a Latin poem, *Elegies against Drunkeness,* written probably by EOBANUS HESSUS attracted much attention (EOBANUS had studied medicine but never achieved his doctor's degree, possibly because of financial reasons. He later became professor of Latin and history in Erfurt and Marburg but, having early become a chronic alcoholic, was merely tolerated with pity). In his book *Bona Valetudinis Conservandae Praecepta* (The rules for keeping in good health) EOBANUS further discussed the dangers of alcohol abuse. In 1518 HEINRICH STROMER VON AUERBACH, professor of medicine in Leipzig published a pamphlet[12] on the serious medical problem of alcoholism, writing that wine might decrease anger, make a person free emotionally and clear a person's thinking but that intoxication and chronic abuse would damage the brain and other organs. He mentioned the dulling of sensations and emotions, of memory and clearness of thinking and the occurrence of damage to the liver, of edema and ascites, of early aging and death. He warned strongly against giving alcoholic beverages to children. The moral and social decline was stressed by him as it was done also by leading humanists.

STROMER's *Decreta* became the basis for a Leipzig dissertation by PFEYL (Leipzig 1531). The student reviewed all the points mentioned by STROMER. It is not an original contribution but drew renewed attention to the problem and to his teacher's book which appeared in the same year. In this period interest in maintenance of health and prevention of illness became widespread in the medical schools. Alcoholism became recognized as a medical-social problem. CORONARO and Italian and French physicians had warned against intoxication from wine. The authors from the northern medical schools (Seidel, Pictorius, Gazabar, Guarinonius) recognized the social as well as the individual problems and by the end of the 16th century the leading textbooks of medicine in-

---

12   HENRICUS STROEMER, *Decreta medica de ebrietate,* Leipzig 1517.

cluded discussion of alcoholism[13, 14]. The publication of well-documented observations attracted attention, especially those by HORST and ROLFINCK. Both described deliria from alcohol which correspond to delirium tremens. SEIDEL wrote that with intoxication vision and hearing are affected and 'manifest hallucinations' may appear. In the chronic state depressive and euphoric features are mentioned as well as deterioration of memory and of behavior.

It is somewhat surprising that dissertations on alcoholism offer few new facts and deal mostly with the elaborations of the condensed statements found in textbooks or with generalities. Alcoholism, usually under the term 'ebrietas' was discussed by a few authors of the 17th century. They offer little of interest except a better differentiation between ebrietas, a voluntary insanity with physical depravation from excessive and unwise consumption of spirituous drinks, and temulentia or frequent intoxication. Brandy or aqua vitae are recognized to be more damaging than beer which, however, was stronger than wine. A good orientation of the literature can be obtained in some dissertations (e.g. KURTZ, Erfurt 1741).

Before 1650 alcoholism is discussed in two dissertations (PFEYL, Leipzig 1531, and MONTIGNY, Paris 1698). In the second part of the 17th century five dissertations deal with this topic (PASOR, Groningen 1653; SUESS, Strasbourg 1656; HANNEMANN, Kiel 1679; WEIDLER, Jena 1689; BREYER, Tübingen 1695). While in the first half of the 18th century 14 dissertations are in our list (GLADBACH, Erfurt 1701; MALLINKROTT, Utrecht 1723; BATTUS, Greifswald 1733; LANGUIS, Wittenberg 1734; PAPEN, Göttingen 1735; MAJAULT, Paris 1737; GÖHRS, Halle 1737; KELLER, Wittenberg 1738; SHERWOOD, Leyden 1739; LUTHERITIUS, Frankfurt a. O. 1740; KURTZ, Erfurt 1741; NAUHEIM, Erfurt 1741; MILLER, Leyden 1743; BECK, Heidelberg 1746). Some of these dissertations reveal the interest of the professors (STENTZEL in Wittenberg, ALBERTI in Halle, and GAUB in Leyden) in this serious medico-social problem which continued to be present to a disturbing degree at many universities. No dissertation appeared from Basel. In the 16th and 17th centuries drinking was excessive in most German universities, frequently by students as well as professors. There was a considerable decrease at the end of the 17th century and in general, the behavior of the students improved. It is

13 OSKAR DIETHELM, *Chronic Alcoholism of Northern Europe.* Akt. Fragen Psychiat. Neurol., vol. 2, p. 29 (1965).
14 BAUER, *op. cit.*

possible that the increase of dissertations on alcoholism is to a considerable extent related to a change in cultural attitude.

The social factors were stressed occasionally. GÖHRS (Halle 1737) might be quoted because he reviewed the alcoholism of women whose behavior in an intoxicated state, and social depravation had distressed the physicians of the 16th and 17th centuries. The question whether or not alcoholic intoxication might affect a fetus and the mother milk was raised repeatedly. Temperance was urged and considered necessary for maintaining good health.

In the 17th century the pharmacologically desirable effect of alcohol was reviewed repeatedly but with no relationship to psychiatric aspects. A considerable group of dissertations dealt in a general way with the effect of alcoholic beverages on health. The superiority of some local beverage became the center of several dissertations – in Paris the good features of wine, in German universities of beer. PRETTENUS (Jena 1684) quotes literature freely to support his theory of the superiority of the beer of his home town because of the special virtue of the water in that region. Similar discussions occurred in the medical literature of the present century.

This chapter which opened with the pamphlet of STROMER VON AUERBACH, can be closed with a discussion (in German) by DEPRÉ (1723)[15] an influential teacher at Erfurt under whose direction a large number of dissertations appeared. Brandy strengthens a person and helps his digestion and is recommended for depressed and hypochondriacal patients. It should not be used in tuberculosis, podagra and mania, and especially avoided in children and woman. The only psychopathological feature he mentioned is poor memory and a reference that under the influence of brandy one becomes easily irritable and angry. The increase of knowledge of alcoholism during two hundred years was apparently not considerable.

5. Opium Addiction

Despite the facts that many foreign and indigenous plants were used to excess there is little in medical literature about psychopathological complications except delirious reactions and brief excitements in connec-

15 JOHANN FRIEDRICH DEPRÉ, *Vom Brauch und Missbrauch des Brandte Weins*, Leipzig 1723.

tion with alkaloids. A dissertation by BOEHMER (Halle 1744), which presents a case of opium addiction, deserves to be quoted. He describes the case of a 50-year-old woman who, since youth, had suffered from a sleep disorder. After the death of her parents (in adolescence) she developed a depression with anxiety and insomnia and received opium. The amount had to be increased and the patient was often slightly stuporous. At 21 she was dependent on opium; menstruation ceased and she became irritable, often frightened. She continued for several years to take 60 grammes of opium daily. Her uneasiness and restlessness persisted; she was tense, had tremors, sometimes she felt as if 'volatile fire, or melted ice' was flowing in her veins. Her torment bent her body into a crooked arc. Her intestines felt as if they were splitting open. When she took opium all these symptoms subsided. She developed marked constipation and bowel movements occurred only with the help of an enema. The physician made the diagnosis of hypochondriaco-hysterical illness. He emphasized that the opium was given for hysterical symptoms which were helped temporarily but then increased. The dosage for adults should vary from 1 to 5 grammes a day and the excessive amount which the patient needed indicated a habit. In different climates, e.g., Persia, much higher amounts could be taken without danger of addiction.

Addiction to opium and to other drugs did not play an important role in European countries. JONES (1700)[16] described toxic conditions which he compared to acute and chronic alcoholism. Drug addiction was known in isolated individual cases, but as a social problem it was not yet recognized or anticipated.

16   JOHN JONES, *The Mysteries of Opium*, London 1700.

Chapter VIII
Psychopathology and Cultural Factors
Psychology, Psychotherapy, Psychopathology

The influence of the cultural factors of the environment, including attitudes of family and community to psychopathologic disturbances, general education, customs and current beliefs and philosophies, are still little understood. It is difficult for a psychiatrist of any given period to recognize these manifold influences, and much more difficult when he tries to understand them by studying the meager literature of the 16th and 17th centuries. Through the centuries, symptoms of psychiatric illnesses changed considerably, frequently to the degree that one does not seem to be dealing with the same illness. Cultural factors affect some symptoms more readily than others. Their effect can be recognized in some dissertations. In the field of psychopathology, which is the science of abnormal mental functions, the influence of humoral pathology extended into the teaching of the 18th century when already chemical and physical concepts had forced the formation of new theories of pathology. Scientific development was hindered by the adherence to rigid scholasticism in some universities, while in others an equally rigid rejection of past theories interfered with scientific curiosity.

1. Psychology

In medical teaching mental functions have been presented according to ARISTOTLE's psychology and its modification by later authors. Arabian and scholastic medicine continued this attitude but, with the early printing (1486) of *De anima,* the physician of the Renaissance had an opportunity to turn to the original source. Medical interest in the relationship of mental and physical functions became manifest in early dissertations.

The textbook of SENNERT[1] together with his book on natural philosophy, seems to have been influential on the teaching of psychology in

1   SENNERT, *o. omnia.*

medicine. SENNERT tried to combine GALEN with the chemical teaching of PARACELSUS, also quoting in his writings many authors of the Renaissance. He presented the rational soul in the Aristotalian meaning. Intelligence and volition are stressed while the emotions received little attention. The 'intellective faculty ... abstracts things from their matter ... It reflects upon itself and knows itself and understands that it does understand'. For such an understanding the help of phantasy is needed which is included in the internal senses. He emphasized the importance of apprehension and cognition, abstraction and judgment. The sensitive soul consists of the external and internal senses. They include the sensus communis, imagination and memory. The later faculty perceives and repeats what has been presented. In man memory has, in addition, the faculty to remember, selecting from a large presentation the material which has been perceived previously and had been forgotten. Dreams are related to imagination.

The small book, *De natura* (1612) by the influential teacher, GREGOR HORST[2] is based on exertia of his medical students and offers a good insight into his teaching. His psychological and psychopathological interests are expressed in the dissertations and exercitia which are referred to under the respective topics. A friend of SENNERT, TOBIAS KNOBLOCH[2] who also taught in Wittenberg, published in 1622 a book which contained a series of disputations. His psychological questions to the students refer to phanthasy, memory, intelligence, dreams in children and in melancholia.

Dissertations which are of interest for obtaining an understanding of the relationship of psychology and medicine include TESSERARIUS (Strasbourg 1626), who appreciated the need to apply psychological knowledge to psychopathology, e.g., demonology. RHOENIUS' analysis (Leipzig 1699) of ARISTOTLE's *De anima* illustrates the long struggle it took medicine to become free from scholastic influence which permitted a new understanding of ARISTOTLE.

The Relationship of Body and Soul

Galenic thinking persisted during the beginning of the 17th century. As late as 1660 GEISSENDÖRFFER (Basel) formulated GALEN's concept

2   HORST, *op. cit.;* KNOBLOCH, *op. cit.*

of the faculties of the senses, movement, imagination, reasoning and memory as the psychological basis for mental illnesses. Like other dissertations before his own it does not make a contribution to an increased understanding of psychopathology. Shortly after DESCARTES' publication[3] appeared its influence became obvious in medical dissertations. His concept of the mind-body dualism remained dominant until a new concept, the unit of mind and body was proposed by STAHL. This author exerted a considerable influence during the 18th century in some of the universities of Germany and in Montpellier.

The theory of DESCARTES appealed to the teachers of the 16th and 17th centuries when the interest centered on obtaining and utilizing in clinical medicine increased medical knowledge whether it be along mechanistic or chemical lines. Dissertations during this period emphasized the importance of emotions on physiological functions, of brain damage on general intelligence, especially memory, and to a small extent on emotions.

A new approach to obtaining an understanding of the relationship of body and mind was offered by the formulation of GEORG ERNST STAHL, the second professor of medicine in Halle. A driving force which he called soul keeps the body in constant motion. The soul forms the body and keeps it in good health, through movements removing that which is disturbing and causing illness. Belief in the self-healing tendency affects STAHL's therapeutic attitude. Psychiatric illnesses are caused by the inhibition of the movements of the soul. While still teaching in Jena he expressed these thoughts in a publication (Diss. epistolica ad ADR. SLEVOGT), *De motu tonico vitali*, Jena 1692. All processes are united in the whole organism. Thus, he replaces DESCARTES' dualism by a concept which in the early 20th century was called the psychobiological unit, the personality. He introduced the dynamic principle to physiologic and psychologic functions, and replaced the concepts of pneuma and animal spirits. The material relationship of emotions and the body is fully presented in the dissertation of REICH (Halle 1695) in which for the first time STAHL's new theories with regard to the relationship of body and mind were presented. It is difficult to state whether some dissertations under the presidium of STAHL were written by the professor or the student. His influence was certainly keenly felt. At other times he wrote an introduction (proempticon) to dissertations, using this oppor-

3   RENÉ DESCARTES, *De homine*, 1662.

tunity to publish new theories[4]. In later years STAHL referred to some students' dissertations as his own publication[5].

REICH's dissertation, on the many kinds of influence of emotions on the human body, presents STAHL's theories which had not been formulated previously in print although they may have been discussed in his lectures to students. He starts with the statement that emotional tranquility is essential for health.

'All vital, animal and rational processes have their basis in the most beautiful harmony and in their indissolvable connection with the force of life [vigor].'

Emotions may cause many changes in the body, including illnesses and pathological signs. Constitutional dispositions which GALEN attributed to the physical structure may change during a person's life, e.g., a dominant emotion may be put into a secondary or lesser position through new emotional habits. Temperament is inborn but becomes modified during life. Emotions which are evoked from within the person, may be the remote and mediate causes of illnesses while emotions related to the impression of external objects are the immediate causes. The Galenic concept that there is a fixed relationship between temperament and definite illness is rejected. All emotions contain a desire for satisfying a goal which is to be united with the external object, to reject it or to escape from it. Strong sensory experiences rarely affect health except if strong emotions are evoked. The suppression of strong emotions by opposite emotions is especially dangerous. The author gives examples of the effect of unusually strong anger, sadness, fear and terror. Interesting

4   Such a proempticon did not need to have a relationship to the student's topic. Other professors used the same procedure to publish comments and discussion on any topic which interested them when a dissertation was published under their praesidium. Sometimes also the dean or the rector used the opportunity in this way. In a proempticon (1965) STAHL discussed synergy; i.e., the working together of nature and medicine, and energy, i.e., self-healing through nature without medical aid. In another proempticon to a dissertation (Halle 1703), he reviewed a physician's visit to a patient's home (De visitatione aegrorum). It is a fine presentation of medical practice and ethics.

5   It was not until 1705 that STAHL gave a complete presentation of his theories in his book Theoria medica vera. REICH's dissertation was translated into German by B. J. GOTTLIEB (1961). This small book also includes a discussion of patient-physician relationship. In contrast to STAHL's theoretical discussions this last publication is very readable and must have influenced the students even if they rejected his theories and preferred to follow the mechanistic concept of FRIEDRICH HOFMANN, the senior professor of medicine in Halle.

observations from literature are given, e.g., that anger and jealousy may cause miscarriage. The physician must consider the role of emotions. Medicines taken in a state of confidence and hope are more effective than if taken in a state of anger or under duress. Injuries to the body may cause severe and chronic emotional illnesses. They can be cured through the healing of the physical damage. Nobody who does not know his own emotional life can understand that of a patient.

SCHMIDT (Halle 1708) made STAHL'steaching the basis for a review of psychopathology. He discussed anxiety, depression, fear and anger and their effects physically and psychologically, acute deliria, mania and melancholia hypochondriaca. The application of STAHL's theories to 'turbulent ideas' and to imagined diseases in hypochondriacal depressions are a brigde to modern psychiatric thinking, as well as the stress on psychotherapy and the avoidance of restraint. Another student of STAHL, WARDENBURG (Halle 1719), studied the effect of large hemorrhages, including the relationship to delirious reactions. The dissertation of DONZELINA (Halle 1714) is not psychiatrically important but might be mentioned because the student presents his teacher's (Prof. STAHL) theories of organism and mechanism. The vital force in the body is strong and able to adapt. Those forces are goal directed[6].

The reaction to STAHL's psychological theories was instantaneous. FRIEDRICH HOFFMANN wrote a proempticon, *De animae et corporis commercio* to HOFSTETTER's dissertation *(De somnambulatione,* Dec. 1695) in which he defended GALEN, stressing that emotions and psychological habits follow the temperaments of the body, and supported DESCARTES' psycho-physical dualism. His student, STANGIUS (Halle 1700) offered a good psychopathological discussion as basis for his teacher's concept of psychiatric illnesses and treatment.

Considering the fundamental and persistent opposition of these two professors it is interesting to read the dissertation of BOROSNYAI (Halle 1728), dedicated to HOFFMANN, who presented clearly the mechanistic concept of his teacher and that of STAHL. It is a sound presentation of opposing viewpoints which speaks well for the freedom of teaching and learning at the university of Halle.

For many readers the concept of 'soul' may be difficult to understand. 'Soul' in the medical dissertations usually meant the principle of life, and infrequently the principle of thought and action, contrasting the

6   STAHL, *op. cit.*

spiritual versus the purely physical. In the present century, European, especially German psychiatry used this term to include all psychological functions. The metaphysical concept of soul, in which the soul is not related to the body is excluded. The psychiatrists who were interested in these considerations were following BERGSON's philosophy of life or the neo-romanticism of KLAGES[7].

The study of man included past as well as combined functions and the whole man. Separate emotions were singled out in the facial expression, in the movements of the body, and in words and sounds, but more frequently the behavior of the whole personality was studied. In the Renaissance when painting and sculpture depicted the human personality and revealed emotions and characteristic behavior, physiognomy flourished. It maintained a moderate influence in the 17th and 18th centuries and began to make a marked impact again at the end of the 18th century, stimulated by the books of LAVATER and to a lesser extent in the present century under the influence of the neo-romantic group. In all these developments the leading principles were the concepts of dynamism and of the whole personality.

It is interesting to note that medical dissertations have rarely dealt with physiognomy. There is, however, a tract on palmistry by a Marburg medical student, GOCLENIUS (1597), which received much attention in some medical groups. This author, later a professor medicine in Marburg, was an influential follower of PARACELSUS and an exponent of his mystical concepts.

Astrology, the science of the influence of the stars on man, was related to Galenic medicine and a guiding principle for prognosis and treatment. Twoards the end of the 16th century some leading physicians questioned the value of astrology, while others, trying to understand the place of man in the cosmos, accepted the influence of the stars[8]; for instance, GOCLENIUS and his pupil ROLFINCK, the influential teacher of Jena. In his consultationes, the latter discussed a patient 'whose parents were astrologically melancholic'. His student MALET (Jena 1696), presenting a patient of 'cold and humid temperament' writes that 'he was born during a very unfortunate constellation of the stars'.

---

7   LUDWIG KLAGES, *Grundlagen der Charakterkunde,* Leipzig 1926.
8   FRANZ ANTON MESMER, in his inaugural dissertation, *De planetarum influxu* (Wien 1766), uses the term in a different meaning, referring to the influence of the atmosphere.

SALZMAN (Strasbourg 1619) rejected the excessive claims and abuses of astromantia. A broader discussion is found in a philosophical dissertation (ENGELBRECHT, Königsberg 1691) which reviewed critically the literature on chiromancy and physiognomy. He included them in the natural type of divination as opposed to spiritual (offered by the prophets and the Church), popular (prediction of farmers on the occurrence of natural phenomena) and diabolical divination. SUPPRIAN (Greifswald 1745) defended physiognomy as the science of diagnosing the learnings of the soul from the organs of the body. Strivings in the body are expressed in one's face, and recognized especially in the eyes and the voice, and secondarily in the cardial response. Through physiognomy it is possible to study critically all mental illnesses. It is interesting to note the change from ENGELBRECHT's concepts of divination to SUPPRIAN's which reveals the increased physiological knowledge and the direction in this development towards LAVATER's concept of physiognomy.

Emotions

The understanding of emotions has always been of interest to physicians and increasingly so with the progress of medicine. Emotions can be observed in the behavior of a person, including their effect on physiological functions and on other persons. Dissertations are cited below to illustrate the trends in evaluating the meaning of emotions and their significance in the study and treatment in clinical medicine.

SCHIFFMANN (Strasbourg 1598), following GALEN's teaching discussed emotions and, influenced by the thinking of the Renaissance, singled out love, greed, sadness, irritability and furor. Quoting GALEN he emphasized the strong effect of emotions on the body, even causing death.

During the 17th century the interest of physicians became increasingly stimulated by the emotions with which they became confronted in psychopathological disorders. The role of emotions in physical illnesses was recognized.

ALBECK's dissertation (Tübingen 1688) illustrates the change which has occurred in the attitutde of physicians to psychopathological disorders and to the significance of delusions. He discusses at length the illness of a 34-year-old woman who asked for help for anxiety, sadness, and fear of some imminent evil, sighing and frequent weeping. The symptoms occurred in paroxysms lasting briefly or for long periods of time. After having obtained the history, he questioned her carefully about her relationship with her husband and children and any external causes which might torture her. He analyzed the situations in which the various symptoms might occur. He then emphasized that between the paroxysms the patient was slow and morose, and he reached the diagnosis of depression, concluding his discussion by an enumeration of the delusions which might occur in a depressive or schizophrenic illness. His description of behavior and delusions is much more detailed than at the beginning of the 17th century.

Special emotions, among them anger, terror and nostalgia, were frequently discussed at length in textbooks and in medical and philosphical treatises and occasionally in dissertations. HOFFMANN (Basel 1699) distinguished petulance which may easily lead to anger, from anger as such. This emotion leads to injury to oneself and is accompanied by aversion toward others and rejection by them. The injury may be real or imaginary and result in angry excitements (mania furibundi). In psychopathological anger, suspicion and fallacious thinking may occur. CLAVILLART (Montpellier 1744) emphasized that hate of varying strength may be present in anger and intensify it. He dwelled especially on the physical symptoms which may accompany anger, such as nausea, vomiting, diarrhea, abdominal cramps and headache. These symptoms may provoke secondary anxiety. As strong emotions weaken the body, medication which decreases the emotion is indicated. Intense anger may also affect the nervous system and the brain. ECKARD (Jena 1697) discussed the symptoms which accompany terror, including seeing ghosts. Terror was frequently found in delirium and melancholia and aggravated physical illnesses. The occurrence of terror in epilepsy may lead to epileptic excitements. TACKIUS (Giessen 1707) reviewed the psychopathology of homesickness which had been first described in the dissertation of HOFER (1688). He described the case of a student of law, a man of delicate constitution and 'lenient education' and of melancholic temperament. When he came from Thüringen to Giessen he seemed constantly sad and developed precordial anxiety accompanied by feeling hot and cold. His appetite became poor, his sleep disturbed and he felt weak. The physician, called in the middle of the night, found the patient sighing, breathing deeply and expressing marked anxiety, which he located in the cardiac region. The symptoms were relieved by carminatives, antapoplectics, anodynes, induced vomiting and laxatives. When, after improvement, the illness returned, the physician asked the patient if his country and parents were always on his mind. This was affirmed. The author considered the patient a dependent and immature person. He was inclined rather to attribute this emotional reaction to insufficient maturity than to accept the Swiss explanation that the change from high to much lower altitudes caused the anxiety.

A great change in the study of emotions occurred around the beginning of the 18th century. VOGHTER (1703) distinguished between the relatively slow, mild and longer lasting effect of worries and depressive moods and the acute, intense and briefer emotions of terror, anger and hate. All these emotional reactions are accompanied by anxiety and apprehension. He reviewed in detail facial expression, tears, sighing, changes in respiration and pulse, and the effect on menstruation. Continued fear and anger may lead to peculiar mental and motor symptoms. Based on STAHL's theories he stressed that basic changes in the body result from emotions and that the cure has to be in a change in the soul, that is through psychotherapy. SEELMAN (Helmstadt 1719), basing his dissertation on chemiatric theories, came to the conclusion that only chemical treatment could be helpful. SCHAEFFER (Rostock 1724) postulated that control of severe and persistent emotions by reason prolongs life. One should judge which emotions are desirable but also recognize the intentions which are directed by emotions. Moderation of emotions can be obtained through education, music and medicine. Early recognition of emotions prevents them from reaching a dominant role. In his final rule of emotional health he urged physicians to recognize emotions which in them produce bias and an uncritical attitude. This dissertation shows the influence of the age of reason and demonstrates also that in practical application the iatrochemists and the followers of STAHL were not always far apart.

CHOMEL (Paris 1731) came to the conclusions that abnormal intensity and duration of emotions damage physical health. SCHAW (Edinburgh 1735), under the influence of BOERHAAVE's teaching and contemporary English philosophy, reviewed abnormal psychological reactions and emotions and their effect on physical illnesses. In several dissertations from Basel (HANHART 1736, LUPICHIUS 1738, STEINER 1739), various aspects of the psychopathology of emotions were studied. HANHART emphasized the importance of the inherent drive in an emotion and of the recognition of proper and mixed emotions. In sad emotions, for instance, fear, anxiety, shame and guilt, terror, horror or desperation may be present. The physiological symptoms vary accordingly. HANHART follows the psychology of CHRISTIAN WOLFF[9]. LUPICHIUS, after a detailed review of literature, discusses the significance of laughter of various types and degrees in physical and psychiatric illnesses. STEINER follows BOERHAAVE's concept of anxiety and recommends his chemical therapy[10]. He mentions, however, that anxiety may be caused by a disturbed conscience and advice from the physician is then indicated but should be combined with physical treatment.

These illustrations demonstrate that in the medical schools of Germany, Basel, Leyden, Utrecht, Edinburgh, and France the psychopathology of emotions was considered important in the study and treatment of patients, whatever theory of the relationship of body and soul was accepted. The result, largely related to contemporary psychology and philosophy, was better medical observation in illnesses and in daily life.

2. Psychotherapy

Psychotherapy, under the influence of STAHL who affected followers and adversaries, began to take on a more critical form than previously. SÜSSENBACH (Halle 1721), using STAHL's concept of far-reaching influence of emotions and related imaginations on the body, discusses the 'imaginary' aspect in treatment and the valuable effect of placeboes. In psychiatric, as well as in physical, illnesses, transient or even lasting beneficial results may be obtained. During temporary relief from anxiety which could increase the pain, the patient's physical recovery may be hastened. The wise physician may make use of current superstitions which cause the patient to expect certain results. Physicians may condemn such teaching as fantastic but use it unknowingly. The author mentioned the importance of the impressions of early childhood, a point which had already been made, but not elaborated upon, by FELIX PLATTER. In the therapeutic procedure, pessimistic attitudes should be changed and the will to live stimulated. Influencing the patient by fear is to be condemned. The therapeutic procedure must be subtle and use, what we now call suggestions. The physiological effect of emotions should be explained and the expectation of certain results introduced. Physical support of psychotherapy by means of diet and a desirable daily routine is indicated. This therapy has been found effective in controlling vomiting

9   CHRISTIAN WOLFF (1679–1754) was professor of philosophy in Halle.
10   BOERHAAVE, op. cit.

and in affecting excretion and bowel movements, in hysteria, hypochondriasis and melancholia. The author offers examples from great physicians of the 16th and 17th centuries which illustrate the far-reaching effect of imagination. Treatments which were recommended by FLUDD and others in the sympathetic cures and by authors of the 17th and 18th centuries in the use of amulets were in this dissertation explained by the use of imagination.

This dissertation on the effect of emotions on the body is far more inclusive than those of other authors who urge its use therapeutically, following the teaching of Leyden (VAN DER HOGBEN, 1715) or Basel where HEGNER (1733) in the treatment of insomnia urges the reduction of disturbing imaginations with their accompanying emotions of sadness, anger and terror.

3. Psychopathology

Aside from the above discussed emotions psychopathology received limited attention in dissertations except in topics dealing with demonology and superstition. Hallucinations in the visual field, frequently related to folklore, and superstitions were reviewed in a few dissertations while delusions and auditory hallucinations were merely mentioned in connection with other clinical topics.

Hallucinations. A common myth which still exists in the rural districts of many European countries is the existence of ghosts and spectres. The appearance of a dead person may be frightening or comforting, dependent on the person's emotional state and on his relationship to the dead person. Other apparitions may relate to one's religious needs or to guilt feelings and expected dreaded punishment. The visual and auditory hallucinations in states of ecstasy have been previously discussed (chap. V). This knowledge of the causative relationship of emotion to hallucinations did not exist in the period under discussion when it was assumed that the ghosts caused the terror. GLYTZ (Jena 1682) presents the case of

‘a 19-year-old man, of melancholic-phlegmatic temperament and a lunatic constitution who was afflicted for some time with a luetic skin condition. One evening when he was waiting on his master he was seized and saw a ghost in the meadow. He was struck by a horror and fear that was worse than panic. Soon he felt with the greatest anguish the weight of the spector itself weighing on him, pressing on his shoulders. He was carried back into the house in a wretched and near lifeless state. He was shuddering and covered with a cold sweat and had lost most of his strength. For two weeks ha had no appetite. Not long afterwards the ghost, recognizable by the same appearance as before, appeared to him, sat down on his bed and seemed to be trying to pull a toe off his right foot. The next day the toe was inflamed and suppurating. There followed shortly violent convulsions and nervous transports, so that he would at one moment bend his body upwards like a bow and then roll up into a ball. He would bite his tongue and this behavior would be accompanied by a higher temperature, more rapid pulse, thirst and constipation. He would sometimes lose the power of speech and sometimes talk deliriously, even threatening to throw himself out of a window. This paroxysm returned periodically. He could even predict its return by the rising of a certain sensation from the lower to the upper parts of his back.'

GLYTZ states the effects of the terror from the sight of the ghost seriously imbalanced the spirits, the nerves and the lymph. He mentioned that it is evident from cases of epileptics that terror has the power to move the animal spirits. WEDEL (Jena 1693) devoted the whole dissertation to a definition that 'spectres are fictitious representations, against the laws of nature, with intact senses, caused by Satanic illusion'. He mentioned folklore and superstition in Thüringen, the wooded mountainous country-side close to Jena, and the literature on elves and other mysterious apparitions. The 2nd part of the dissertation dealt with the effect of apparitions.

In fever or under the influence of alcoholic beverages specters may appear and frighten the patient, resulting in convulsions (they may be epileptic or hysterical in character). STRUVIUS (Halle 1725) reviewed the literature on ghosts, citing ridiculous and fabulous observations by prominent medical and legal authorities of past centuries, including the publications of TANDLER, KIRCHMAJER and WEDEL. He also gave considerable space to theologic authors who had supported the existence of some apparitions on a religious basis. This interesting dissertation is to a large extent devoted to demonology and superstition. From a psychopathological point of view he explained these visions as errors of phantasy under the influence of terror, fear, anxiety, or related to a damage of the sensory organ, or mental illness. Contributing factors are ignorance and frequently deceptions. Imobility when perceiving a ghost is caused by horror. Reference is also made to a physical explanation of apparitions in some mountainous regions which might be related to metals in the rocks (this formulation was presented by RUDOLF WILHELM CRAUSIUS in a proempticon to the dissertation of PH. W. STOCKHAUSEN, Jena 1712).

In connection with these discussions on spectres it is pertinent to refer to the dissertation by LEVIN (Halle 1740) who from a Stahlian point of view discussed the relationship of phantasy, sensorium commune and memory. He clearly separated sensations and imagination and rejected the localization of imagination as it had been postulated by VAN HELMONT, DESCARTES and WILLIS. He accepted that imagination can have a far-reaching influence on physiologic manifestations and illnesses but stressed there were definite limitations, e.g., imagination could not affect the fetus, resulting in abnormalities of the newborn child. The occurrence of anaesthesia under various conditions was studied by QUISTORP (Rostock 1718). With intact memory, imagination and sensus communis, the absence of sensations in the whole body, with the exception of the vital sensation, had been observed. He mentioned that the highest degree of anaesthesia would be found in catalepsy, less in ecstasy and lethargy, and little with fainting and deep meditation. Anaesthesia might occur under torture but is not caused by something magic.

Chapter IX
Psychopathology and Cultural Factors
Demonology, Superstition and Treatment

During medieval times the power of the devil became of increasing concern to people, educated and uneducated. It was accepted that this power of evil was possible by the permission of God. The belief of theologians and jurists that human beings were in league with the devil to receive powers in exchange for their souls was adopted. The power of magicians and witches was greatly feared and admired in the 15th century and also became increasingly linked with heresy. Towards the end of the century this fear and the cruel prosection of witches resulted in psychic epidemics, the full nature of which is still unclear[1]. The power of the alchemist frightened people, and scientists like AGRIPPA of NETTESHEIM and many others of lesser stature were eyed suspiciously. Mentally sick patients, suffering from schizophrenia, depressions, senility, hysterical and other psychopathological reactions developed symptoms which were considered daemonomania. A frightened and persecuted populace reacted with aggression against unfortunate patients, and others they accused of being under demonological influence. At some universities it was taught in the 16th century that it was at times true that witches could fly to their magic Sabbaths where they danced, dined and performed remarkable deeds. They had sexual intercourse with the devil. Witches had the power to stir up tempests, storms, thunder, calms, fog, hailstorms, snowstorms, corrupt water and air; they sprinkle dust in the air from which locusts, caterpillars and various insects harmful to fruit are born, and produce mice which destroy growing things, spiders and butterflies, but not the more perfect animals like cows and camels, and make brute animals talk, and fascinate them, starve them, enchant them, snatch away infants and leave changelings in their place. Witches enticed men to sexual perversions, caused sterility in men and women and male impotency. In the 15th century sorcerers and witches were declared heretics and condemned to death by burning. Torture became the accepted tool to obtain confessions. With the reformation, these beliefs

1   HECKER, *op. cit.*

and cruel practices were espoused by both Churches in the search and punishment of heretics and witches.

Scholars, including physicians, attacked demonology but frequently accepted the power of the devil. The books on this topic which have contributed much to the change of attitude among physicians as well as books by theologians and jurists have to be read in their entirety in order to be able to understand the slow progress to an enlightened attitude during the 17th century. The psychiatric and general medical and social aspects are still bewildering to the modern reader. It may be difficult to recognize the Arabic influence and that of the Greek and Roman writers in the context of 15th and 16th century philosophy and theology, and the superstitious and suggestive influences of the existing cultures.

A few of the great medical writers of this period may be quoted to illustrate the influences to which the teachers and students of medicine were exposed – at a period when medicine was not only the art of restoring health but also that of preserving it. The previously quoted GUAI-NERIO († 1450)[2] questioned the statement of the Arabic authors[3] that through the influence of demons 'certain melancholic persons foretold the future and that their predictions came to pass, and some others who were illiterate became literate to the point that in certain fields of learning they undertake discussion on a proposition and reply to objections'. He also attacked the argument that there are two ways of acquiring knowledge, one through discursive reasoning and teaching, the other through celestial influence. GUAINERIO closed his lengthy discussion with 'I relinquish to theoreticians, and I pass on to the glories of practice'[4]. FERNEL (1497–1558) accepted the influence of the occult and that nature might be interfered with by magical forces, 'the work of evil men imitating, by means of demons, the divine'. Possessed persons might re-

2   GUAINERIUS, op. cit.
3   The Greek physicians recognized a divine influence.
4   Another point of view is presented by LANGE, op. cit., epistola XXXIV:
'In 1554 in Rome some 45 women, some of them widows, obsessed by demons, while being led to an exorcism at the altar ... went insane in church, incredible as it may seem, like the priests of Cybele and with a terrible voice began wailing and fell on the ground as if they were dead, and dashed their heads against the walls and the floor, without however any injury. It is horrible to relate with what trembling voices they responded in Latin to the questions of the presiding bishops and other officials, even though they were illiterate, and with what lamentable voices, afflicted with the fierce torments of the sick, they wailed.'
LANGE states that medicine may be helpful for some of the somatic symptoms accompanying possession but that only the exorcist can effect a cure.

semble states of mania[5]. With increasing experience and knowledge FERNEL recognized many superstitions and became more critical of astrology and of the untoward influence of the stars on health which he had previously accepted. LEMNIUS (1505–1568)[6], whose book was frequently quoted by medical students of the 16th and 17th centuries, stated 'humors and not bad angels cause diseases, yet the aerial spirits do mix themselves therewith and increase the diseases by adding fire unto them'. This author who accepted many superstitions wrote 'melancoliques, mad and frenzy people, and such as are furious from other causes will sometimes speak strange tongues they never learned and yet not be possessed by the devil'. It was hidden in the mind of man, and influenced humors stir what is hidden. If the symptom is not cured by purging medications nor by opiates producing sleep, it was caused by the devil. WEYER (Wierus) (1515–1588)[7] attacked demonology vigorously and most critically but he did not deny the existence of the devil and possible evil influences on health. In his introductory dedication to the Duke of Cleve he briefly presented his theologic attitude when he stated that his argument would be partly theological, presenting the slyness and zeal of the devil as proven in the sacred writings, and partly philosophical, reflecting with natural reasons the empty mockery by the devil and the corrupt imaginations of so-called witches. Then, he would deal medically with the topic, demonstrating the natural origin of diseases which had been attributed to the power of witches, and finally discuss the legal aspects of punishment. His attitude is not very different from FELIX PLATTER (1536–1613)[8] who accepted a demoniacal influence in a case of distortion of the body (probably torticollis) because he could not explain the symptom on a natural basis (observations, p. 20). These physicians who lived in the stirring, medically and culturally rapidly changing 16th century, must have altered their opinions during their life time and their books do not always reflect their development as is so well demonstrated in SHERRINGTON's study of FERNEL. The last influential teacher of this period of widely accepted demonology who should be mentioned is SENNERT (1572–1637)[9]. He distinguished natural from supernatural dreams by God, good angels and devils. He also recognized a demonia-

5   SHERRINGTON, op. cit.
6   LEMNIUS, op. cit.
7   WEYER, op. cit.
8   PLATTER, op. cit.
9   SENNERT, op. cit.

cal type of sopor which occurred when a witch believed that she had experienced various types of experiences with demons. He accepted that demonological influences might be present in chorea (probably referring to dancing mania). SENNERT, like WEYER and other authors accepted the existence and influence of the demon, but denied the power of witches and sorcerers.

Two Wittenberg professors who wrote on this type were widely quoted. HIERONYMUS NYMAN (1554–1594)[10] in an oratio on imagination (1603) was skeptical of occult action in some drugs in affecting cures, attributing the effect to imagination. However, he believed in the occult faculty of amulets and the diabolical magic effect of weapon ointments. TANDLER (1571–1617)[11], discussing bewitching and incantations, assumes a natural or magic action. He was against many current superstitions but accepted the great power of demons.

Demonology was rarely discussed at length in dissertations of the 16th and 17th centuries but there frequently occur brief references to it. SCHWENCKFELT (Basel 1587) accepted a possible influence of demons in melancholia. FABRI (Tübingen 1593) discussed the medical-theological attitude that demons can cause melancholia and should be healed by prayers and not by drugs. This may occur in simple-minded women. He offered good clinical data of schizophrenic and depressive symptoms which occur on a natural basis. BATTUS (Rostock 1605) denied the existence of demonological causes of melancholia as also did WALTER (Jena 1652) while GERSTMANN (Jena 1652) admitted demonological influence if the patient spoke in a foreign language which he had not learned. These two dissertations are interesting because both were written under the presidium of ROLFINCK. RHENANUS (Marburg 1615) discussed lycanthropy which he did not consider a true change of man into wolf, whereas others stated that through the power of the devil magicians can change into werewolves.

The wolves and wild dogs were feared dangers in the medieval forests and it was not surprising that the Greek metempsychosis, the change of man into a wolf, played a great role in European folklore. Schizophrenic and paranoid patients, believing that they had been changed into dogs or wolves, imitated the behavior of these animals, leaving their homes at night and going about the city, walking on all fours and howling like a wolf until dawn. They were said to visit ceme-

10 NYMANN, op. cit.
11 TANDLER, op. cit.

teries, breaking into graves and stealing bodies, which they carried around on their shoulders. These patients were described as having a pallid complexion, dry and hollow eyes, showed an extraordinary thirst and had sores on their shins caused by their frequent falls. Some of them bit people, like a dog, the disease therefore called cynanthropy. This description, found in Castelli's Lexicon (1721)[12], was probably known to most students and the picture was strengthened by local folklore.

RHENANUS (Marburg 1615) considered it a mere delusion of the patient who believed that he had been changed into a wolf. When he appeared as a wolf to others, this happened through the aid of the devil who fascinated the senses of men. The student offered no clinical material which might help the modern reader to decide whether such a statement might have been based on induced insanity. SCHMILAUER (Wittenberg 1608) included the ecstatics among melancholia; i.e., schizophrenia, and explained that a boy speaking in a foreign tongue used Latin or other foreign words which he had heard, presenting them in a gibberish-like conversation. He accepted, however, that in a melancholia demons might cause this symptom, and that melancholia could be caused by witches. His teacher TANDLER had maintained an opposite point of view.

The influence of the devil on bodily functions was affirmed by LE GAIGNEUR (Paris 1638), while BÜHREN (Erfurt 1698) explained the symptoms by emotions. He saw 'no need to invent the devil'. WAXMANN (Jena 1687) and SOMMER (Jena 1693) expressed themselves more cautiously. It is interesting to note that in 1670 the opinion of the medical faculty of Jena was requested on two sisters who were accused of being witches. Despite a clear medical history of epilepsy, or possibly hysteria, the faculty concluded that it was an 'affectus mixtus', i.e. natural and supernatural.

Ecstasy was frequently observed in religious devotion but critical observers distinguished the purely religious experience from the psychopathological. It is not surprising that the possibility of diabolical ecstasy was often considered, but one is astonished by the strong defence of demonology offered by STOLTERFOHT (Greifswald 1692):

'We see plenty of examples of demoniacs or people possessed by the devil whom we see agitated by the devil in a thousand fashions. At one moment their mouths are twisted; at another we find the devil acting on the body itself and swelling it up.'

12   CASTELLI, *op. cit.*

Dissertations devoted to the topic of demonology appeared in the first quarter of the 18th century when FRIEDRICH HOFFMANN felt the need to clarify the religious, philosophical and medical aspects of demonology. His student (BÜCHING, Halle 1703), after some general questions about the devil's power, affirmed the devil's influence on the human body, via the elements, especially the air, and via the mind.

'It is possible for a person's diet to predispose him to vulnerability to diabolical influence, especially if it creates melancholy. Southern Europeans drink wine and cultivate lively interests which keep melancholy away, and among them one rarely hears of concern with witches, while northern Europeans drink beer and eat coarse food. Among them tales of ghosts and demonism abound.'

Later, this author stated that the devil can control the spirits in the body, and by augmentation produce violent motions, contortions of the body, unnatural strength, convulsions, spasms, and pain. By diminishing the spirits the devil produces sexual impotence and insensibility of the skin. Uterine suffocation, opisthotonus, St. Vitus' Dance, and epilepsy may also be caused by the devil. It is important, however, that one distinguishes diabolically-caused diseases from natural ones. A supernatural cause can be accepted if the following signs are present: Convulsions with no prior symptoms, accompanied by blasphemy, knowledge of future or hidden things, knowledge of languages with which the patient had no contact, unnatural strength of the patient, vomiting of miscellaneous objects like keys, hair, bits of wood or stones or discharging objects from the ear, vagina or penis.

The existence of demonological influence was defended but more frequently rejected by medical publications as well as by dissertations from the theology faculties (i.e. at Tübingen under the praesidium of OSIANDER) and law at German universities. Effective arguments against the acceptance of demonological causes in illnesses and an attack on superstitions in general came from Kiel dissertations where the teachers were greatly influenced by BOYLE's philosophy. BURCHARDUS (Kiel 1704) gave an interesting historical review, including the testimony of magic in sacred books and profane history. He considered the signs of magic illnesses as fallacious and superstitious. His detailed discussion of the use of amulets and parts of the body of animals or human beings and explanation of the therapeutic results through imagination is interesting. Similarly the affect of incantations and of carefully chosen words is presented as what we now call suggestion. This dissertation on magical ef-

fect and treatment by magic was followed a few months later by the one
of LAURENTIUS (Leipzig 1704), initially dealing with the belief of possession by the devil. The persistence of prejudice is well illustrated by the
fact that OHM (Heidelberg 1681) considered it important to state that
neither PARACELSUS nor CORNELIUS AGRIPPA nor TRITHEMIUS was diabolical.

QUISTORP (Rostock 1718), as mentioned previously, discussed the
various psychopathological conditions in which a patient might not respond to pain or other sensory stimuli. This state might also occur in
physical illness and under torture but never was there an indication of
magical anaesthesia.

FRIEDRICH HOFFMANN, the famous Halle internist, persistently maintained his attitude of possible diabolical influence[13]. In 1723 he gave an
expert opinion to the faculty on a 21-year-old patient who insisted and,
corresponding to the superstition of his time, described in detail a pact
he had made with the devil. His physician made the diagnosis of hypochondriacal melancholia. The judge asked for an opinion of the medical
faculty which analyzed the case well and considered the statements delusional but stated that attempts at seducing a person by the devil must be
accepted. In 1725 HOFFMANN republished BÜCHING's dissertation of
1703, without mentioning the student's name. The title page merely
states that it is an improved edition (emendatio jam edita). The changes,
however, merely consist of a few 'improvements' in Latin. HOFFMANN,
through this edition, gave the great prestige of his name to the support
of demonology, stating that the devil acts through the animal spirits.
This is the medium of his power over witches.

STRUVIUS (Halle 1725) (see p. 21), under the praesidium of ALBERTI
concluded his dissertation with STAHL's natural explanation of visual
hallucinations (ghosts) but leaving it open as to what extent demonic
power might make use of natural functions. Another student of ALBERTI,
CORVINUS (Halle 1725) carefully reviewed the medical literature and
Protestant and Catholic theologians' discussion of demonology. Following his professor's teaching of the body-soul relationship he concluded
that it is possible for the devil, by divine permission, to use natural
forces to produce visions by using an eye which had been damaged by
an illness or causing diseases of the mind as other authors had assumed.
He concludes with the statement nothing can prove or disprove such a
hypothesis.

13   FR. HOFFMANN, Medicina consultatoria, Halle 1721, Dec. II, p. 153.

STEVER (Rostock 1721) in twenty propositions concluded that various illnesses, including melancholia, mania, catalepsy, hysteria, opisthotonus and convulsions were spurious obsessions. In proposition 21 he presented the theological attitude and later disputed the pathognomic signs of true obsession. The dissertation closes with an interesting discussion of treatment.

Fascination, i.e., the influence through a person's eye, has probably interested people throughout the history of mankind. The strong emotions of hate and jealousy, of admiration and love effect persons through facial expressions which have been largely related to the eyes. This expression is poorly described but is even now readily accepted. According to Arabic and Renaissance physicians the eyes were said to have a magic influence, and thus the physician's will can affect a patient – a statement not far removed from the hypnotic technique of the last century. Various physiological explanations have been offered. Supernatural fascination by magicians and witches seems to have been mentioned very little in medical literature. There are some dissertations which might be reviewed. SCHREINER (Tübingen 1633) discussed magic fascination which, according to his widely quoted literature, may cause intense love. DU PRÉ (Paris 1630) denied that fascination can cause emaciation, while DE LARBRE (Paris 1678) and KÄSEBERG (Jena 1682) maintained this possibility. The phenomena which KÄSEBERG described in a young woman were 'beyond the sphere of nature'. He stressed, however, that many diseases which give the impression of witchcraft are due to natural causes, e.g., melancholia, mania, convulsions, sterility of either sex, wasting of the body. An interesting historical review is offered by GENSELIUS (Erfurt 1725) who accepted possible demonological influences in fascination.

The 16th century was characterized by superstition and gullibility which were used by skilled charlatans as well as by conscientious physicians who were convinced of the truth of their theories. Many therapeutic procedures which were sometimes explained by magic influences seem to have been effective through suggestion. While it was still difficult for a TANDLER or HORST to explain on a natural basis such phenomena as fascination and spectres, their questions on these topics seem to have stimulated the students to search for answers. With the progress of science and increased clinical knowledge, critical questioning appeared in literature and teaching. An interesting example of good observation in clinical medicine with critical questioning is the dissertation of

RICHTER (Kiel 1720) who recognized psychological factors in his patient's illness instead of searching for mystical explanations. He presented in considerable length the observations on a Catholic woman who developed a hysterical reaction when she attempted to join the Protestant Church. She was not able 'to eat the body of Christ', became greatly distressed and hated herself. After a few days, convulsions, which she had in church at the age of 25, reappeared. Shortly afterwards her legs became paralyzed and she was unable to control her bladder. Later she became deaf and mute for a period of time. Her paralyzed state lasted six years. One night she had a vision of a man in white who told her to eat. In another vision she was told to have hope. She now noticed the gradual return of sensations in her abdomen and later in her legs. When daylight came she was able to dress and began to walk with support from others. The improvement continued steadily. It is interesting to read the critical discussion by the student, especially the recognition of the psychological factors instead of the searching for a mystical explanations.

Superstitions of many types were important during the three centuries under discussion. It is often difficult to characterize them as mystical as they are based on lack of knowledge, fallacy and culturally established convictions. ALBERTI, a former minister, sought the clarification of demonology and superstition in his religious beliefs and in the psychology of STAHL. The group in Königsberg and Kiel attacked the problem more directly on a medical basis, following the teaching of DE LE BOË and BOYLE. The dissertation of ENGELBRECHT (Königsberg 1691) included an excellent critical review of literature, including the various types of divination, chiromancy, astrology and physiognomy, and of their leaders (FLUDD, JOHANNES AB INDAGINE, GOCLENIUS and NICOLAI POMPEJUS).

The use of amulets as practiced by physicians was less related to demonological or mystical thinking than to ignorance and superstition. Its curative value was confirmed by DU PONT (Paris 1693). After a good review of current superstitions TEUTSCHER (Erfurt 1720) discussed the possible value of therapeutic suggestions made by medical leaders of the preceding two centuries.

The influence of *philters* to obtain power over another person is an interesting example of the use of superstition and empirical knowledge of the effect of some herbs and minerals. In the 16th century PARACELSUS and other chemiatric physicians were attacked for using drugs of magical influence. A critical attitude began to appear in the dissertation by ZOLLIKOFER (Basel 1621) who questioned that it was possible by pharmaceutic means to induce love and sexual drives towards a specific person and he rejected various claims in literature. The attitude of his cultural period is seen in his final statement that the devil, with God's permission, can so deprave the imagination of woman that she can commit the most malicious and horrible acts. Another critical attitude is found in a reference by POLNER (Basel 1632) who mentioned love philters as one of the causes of toxic excitements, including as the dangerous ingredients atropa belladonna and hyoscyamus as well as cat brain. Similar references are found in other dissertations on mania (MATTHIS, Strasbourg 1669; PRINTZ, Jena 1708). CLAUDERUS (Leipzig 1661) reviewed literature carefully, clearly illustrating medical and general superstitions of the 16th and 17th centuries and the occult; i.e., as yet unrecognizable properties in many medicaments, a point which had already been stressed by SENNERT. The medical students VISCHER and TEUTSCHER, in a combined publication (Leipzig 1711) drew the conclusion from their study of literature that in love potions imagination plays an essential role. WOLFF (Wittenberg 1726) considered the aphrodisiac properties in drugs and the propensity to induce ecstatic states (ZORNIUS, Rostock 1707), documenting his discussion with a wealth of references to past and more recent literature. These dissertations illustrate the persistent belief among medical and lay people in the possible or even probable power of drugs to induce sexual stimulation and potency.

The attitude of medicine to *sexual problems* was always bound closely to culture. The dissertations of Paris and Reims are illuminating. Some of them deal with questions which psychiatry still has not been able to answer satisfactorily. The therapeutic use of sexual intercourse in hysteria was still discussed 150 years after the dissertation by CHAUVEL (Paris 1674). To him 'hysterical melancholy is the inseparable compassion of intense burning desire (for the male seed)'. Previously MAURIN (Paris 1658) had affirmed the desirability of sexual intercourse in women suffering from melancholia. The value of sexual intercourse had already been stated by HERNAEUS (Paris 1546) and later by BLUMBERG (Jena 1685) and BLANCHARD (Reims 1690). The fact that sexual desires might cause mental illness was the topic of dissertations of HUBAULT (Paris 1621) and PUYLON (Paris 1630). BUVARD (Paris 1604) and DE QUANTEAL (Paris 1669) stated that sexual desires affect mental faculties. Other discussions dealt with the sexual aspects in hysteria and sexual excitements, and with the abnormal intensity of love which have been discussed in chapters VI and VII. The effect of salaciousness was considered in connection with fecundity (DE MAGNY, Paris 1720), headaches (DU VAL, Paris 1662), fever (GLASEMEYER, Jena 1689; HAGEN, Königsberg 1708; LAMBERTUS, Leyden 1706; MARQUARD, Leyden 1706) and life span (MAURIN, Paris 1657). In the 18th century the love fever was substituted by chlorosis and was a popular topic for dissertations in the 18th and 19th centuries. Physiological, psychological and psychopathological studies of sexual functions progressed little until the end of the 19th century. Scientific development and changes in cultural and social attitudes helped in the advance of knowledge. Male sexuality became of equal interest. In the 17th century dissertations on satyriasis in the psychopathological sense were rare and not very interesting in contrast to those on furor uterinus for which gradually the term, nymphomania, was used. Lasciviousness in men was considered normal and admirable, and the lack of sexual control the male privilege.

Two interesting dissertations are on the topic of chastity. HOFER (Basel 1716) and ZINDEL (Basel 1745) studied the literature on psychopathological and physical reactions to a chaste life in religious orders. In contrast to the statements found in the medical literature of the 19th century they concluded that no ill effects could be attributed to prolonged chastity.

Incubus (ephialtes) had been recognized by the Greek and Latin physicians as a sleep disorder which was caused by impending apoplexy, by epilepsy, mania and indigestion (Aetius, Oribasius). The topic appeared regularly in medical literature but no reputable writer seems to have implied a magical meaning (GERBER, Jena 1653). This statement is supported by our study of fifteen at random selected dissertations on incubus. Incubus had become a medical term for nightmare, the symptom of an underlying physical disorder, emotional distress, and according to some authors also related to hysteria.

Dreams as such were not a topic for dissertations. Occasionally there was reference to them using SENNERT's distinction of natural and supernatural dreams[14]. In dissertations on melancholia, mania and delirious illness fearful dreams were mentioned. Divination was seldom mentioned except in the discussion of magical forces.

Astrology which has been discussed previously (chap. VIII) became of decreasing interest to physicians and lay people during the 17th century.

14 SENNERT, *op. cit.* and *Thirteen books of natural philosophy,* London 1659.

The dissertations dealing with *specters* (ghosts) deserve some mentioning. This superstition was still widespread in the 19th century. Dissertations dealing with ghosts psychopathologically, i.e., studying them as visual hallucinations, are not significant in contrast to those which describe and review the intense fear reactions to seeing a ghost. GLYTZ (Jena 1682), whose case was reviewed on page 127 offered an explanation based on DESCARTES and his own teacher, FRIEDRICH HOFFMANN:

'When the sick man is struck by horror, the qualities (of the spirits) which are stirred up are driven from the circumference to the center and cease fermentation. Hence, stillness of the aether, in which DESCARTES says the cold consists, should necessarily follow.'

The cold sweat is the effect of the lymph. The dissertation by STRUVIUS (Halle 1725) follows the teaching of ALBERTI. He tried to explain the nature of superstition involved, thus offering the reader an insight into the beliefs and folklore of the countryside in Thüringen and other parts of Germany. He described the horror of his patient but without a penetrating analysis. A dissertation by WEDEL (Jena 1693), whose father GEORG WOLFGANG WEDEL in 1691 had written a critical *propempticon de contractura Daemonica,* is based on the definition that ghosts are representations, with intact senses, formed by satanic illusions. He tried to prove his definition by citing experiences of his own and others and by the folklore of the region. He discussed the frequency of this visual hallucination in depressions, fever and alcoholic intoxication. These dissertations are interesting because they are based on different theories and attitudes to superstitions. GEHREN (Rostock 1729) offers a critical review of the superstition of ghosts and how seeing them may cause emotionally precipitated pathological reactions.

Tarantism offers an example of uncritical thinking in medicine. Described briefly but clearly by SENNERT and other authors before him, this endemic and sometimes epidemic illness attracted little attention in literature until it was described at length by the well-known clinician BAGLIVI[15]. His description and explanation were accepted without criticism. This attitude is best illustrated in MEAD's publication (1702)[16] which also reveals a similar uncritical attitude on the effect of the changing phases of the moon on mentally ill people, epilepsy and physical illnesses. The description of tarantism stresses that after having been bitten by a tarantula after a few hours the patient develops a localized inflamma-

15   BAGLIVI, *Opera omnia,* Paris 1788.
16   MEAD, *op. cit.*

tion around the bite, accompanied by violent nausea, difficulty in breathing and faintness. The patient looks depressed and becomes increasingly stupid, timorous and in a short time will expire. If, however, he hears music his arms and legs begin to move and the patient starts to dance. After three to five hours the patient rests and then dances again, this behavior repeating itself until the patient fully recovers. The following summer the symptoms will recur if not prevented by music, and the patient becomes incurable. When dancing the patients behave foolishly and talk and act obscenely. Scorpions may have a similar effect. This illness was observed in summertime in certain parts of Italy and therefore, unknown to the physicians of the northern countries. HÜBNER (Strasbourg 1674) defined the illness as being of occult quality and included the above-mentioned symptoms. He stressed individual differences in the behavior of the patients which were related to different kinds of tarantula. NOËL DE PIVIER (Frankfurt a. O. 1691) also bases his discussion on the older authors, accepting the behavior as a toxic reaction. Psychiatrically, neither dissertation offers much of interest. GOURRAIGNE (Montpellier 1732) confirmed that music was the sole remedy, describing the type of music and instruments that had been found most useful.

Treatment of all psychiatric disorders was discussed fully in most of the dissertations but offered little new. The treatment differed little from that recommended by the pre-Renaissance authors. Evacuation by vomitoria, purgatives, induced sneezing and sweating, blisters and bleeding was considered essential. The drug treatment of the Arabs which included the recommendations of the Greek physicians and plants of their native land was substituted partly by herbs which were indigenous to Europe and by chemical medication. Despite the change in theories no radical modifications were proposed. FERNEL treated by the doctrine of contraries, using herbs and the complicated mithridate and theriac. SENNERT stressed the occult qualities in jewels and rare minerals. (Occult might mean mysterious, supernatural or merely unknown.) RIVIÈRE offered examples of uncritical procedures, often related more to folklore than to science. He mentioned, e.g., in his observations the cure of hysterical fits which imitated epilepsy by the patient wearing a piece of the flesh of a wolf. The tendency to be guided by belief and hope instead of critical reasoning has persisted in medicine, including professors as well as students and graduates. The treatment proposed in the dissertations followed orthodox lines. The authors usually do not define terms which were assumed to be clear but could well have several meanings. The highly praised hippomanus which was claimed to be effective in sexual excitements (LEHMANN, Erfurt 1715) might be a plant found in Arcadia, sweat from the pubic area of a mare, or the skin on the forehead of a newly born foal.

The use of music in the treatment of melancholia has been recommended by the ancient and succeeding authors. During the Renaissance period and in the 17th and 18th centuries the therapeutic value of music was emphasized. HARADUIN DE S. JACQUES (Paris 1624) confirmed its efficacy and JÖCHER (Leipzig 1714) discussed its effect on man in health and illness. Whatever the therapeutic value, the tool used was pleasing and in no way damaging. This cannot be said of another tool, flagellation, which was recommended to make combative and destructive patients amenable to cooperate. Physical punishment was rarely mentioned as desirable but the fear of flogging was considered of therapeutic value. In a brief tract the highly esteemed JOHANN HEINRICH MEIBOM[17], professor in Helmstadt, reviewed in 1659 the ancient authors and those of the Renaissance who had recommended flogging in madness and for sexual stimulation. In the new edition which was edited by his son (1669) THOMAS BARTHOLINUS (Copenhagen) supported the treatment for 'those who dissemble diseases' and for distempers of the body and soul and those who pretend to be possessed. Madness is prevented by the fear of pain. A physician should not be deterred by his horror of this treatment because one should not be guided by whether the treatment gives pain or pleasure but by whether it is helpful or not. No dissertations were devoted to the therapeutic use of flagellation but its need was mentioned for unruly or excited patients. An example is given by SCHROEDER (Erfurt 1695) who mentioned a 25-year-old student of a 'manic-depressive temperament'. Under the pressure of his studies he developed a violent excitement, characterized by anger, truculence, a threatening expression, outbursts of destructiveness and physical aggression. When tied to the bed hand and foot he spit at people and cursed them. Discussing the difficulty of controlling this excitement the author stated:

'Experience teaches that the excessive ferocity of maniacs can be controlled by the use of sticks and clubs. They often ease up at the sight of a menacing club and pretend to lose their wild furor. It is amazing how maniacs fear (these) more than death.'

17   MEIBOM, op. cit.

STEVER (Rostock 1721) referred to the use of flagellation. Fear as a therapeutic tool was re-emphasized repeatedly, e.g. at the beginning of the 19th century and also 30 years ago when some psychiatrist considered fear the essential feature of convulsive therapy.

The use of spas in depressive illnesses, hypochondriasis and other psychoneurotic illnesses had been recommended by ancient and Renaissance writers. Spas became fashionable at the end of the 18th century, highly recommended and publicized by CHEYNE[18] and FRIEDRICH HOFF-MANN. This leading internist wrote several publications on the value of mineral springs, singling out several spas in Germany. Under his guidance students submitted dissertations which are interesting documents of medical naïveté and desire for economic gain. In psychiatry this tendency has been obvious in the recommendation of special foods and drugs from the Renaissance to the present time. The use of amulets, which was discussed above, flourished during past periods of superstition but in various forms has still been considered in modern literature. Blood letting, purging, induced vomiting, selective foods and hypnotics have been in widespread use supported by changing theories. In modern times these trends have been less marked but even in this century, for instance, intensive purging and the use of emetics has been proposed in psychiatric literature and transiently attracted a considerable following.

Psychotherapy, in the form of kind understanding, encouragement, distraction and not recognized suggestions, has been recommended in textbooks and mentioned at various lengths in dissertations. Under the influence of STAHL (chap. VIII) psychotherapy in a modern sense developed at the end of the 17th and 18th centuries.

Preservation of health and prevention of illness began in the 16th century and soon was taught in books and at medical schools. As was mentioned previously (chap. VII), the social problem of alcoholism was studied and medical advice offered. Another important medical-social problem was recognized in the occurrence of suicide. There is little in medical and general literature before 1750 which would indicate a marked increase in suicide. The publication of dissertations may be part of the increased interest in physical and mental health. FRIEDRICH HOFF-MANN (Jena 1681) wrote an interesting and informative dissertation in which he reviewed Greek and Latin medical and philosophical attitudes. He then quoted medical observations of the 18th century and emphasized the depressive features. In discussing the signs which indicate sui-

18   GEORGE CHEYNE, *An essay on regimen*, London 1740.

cidal danger, he mentioned the combination of fearfulness and sadness, solitude and poor sleep, disturbing delusions, despair of God's forgiveness and continuous depression. Among aggravating conditions he included constitutional factors and senility. He also warmed of suicidal danger in some excitements. The means used were poison, self-starvation, hanging and drowning. GLOXIN (Halle 1724) stressed, in addition, the need to be aware of the obvious (violent) and hidden (not recognized) suicidal dangers. He emphasized the uncontrollable emotions such as vehement anger, sadness, desperation, envy and hate, and their danger under influence of alcoholic intoxication. In his accompanying remarks the presiding professor, Alberti, discussed suicides among scholars and litterati.

OBER (Kiel 1701) warned against a lack of appreciation of the strength of imagination which can make physical illnesses worse and cause even death by the effects of resulting terror. If imagination is against the treatment, the cure of an illness is more difficult. The physician's understanding of these factors is important so that he can develop a desirable attitude in treatment. STEGMANN (Halle 1722) critically discussed the attitude of the physician, and how he can use in good conscience the drugs, alcohol and diet which are prescribed. He urged physicians not to treat patients who are psychologically untreatable or do not cooperate, except by supportive psychotherapy and clearly needed physical treatment. Physicians should not find excuses for lack of success by blaming heredity, nor should they treat by means which they know do not help. He quoted STAHL's criticism of the use of the mineral waters from spas, so strongly recommended by HOFFMANN. This dissertation urged a correction and prevention of medical uncritical attitudes and abuses which 20 years later have been so vividly criticized by MOLIÈRE.

In the 18th century *legal medicine* developed rapidly. Among dissertations brief mention is made of legal-psychiatric problems which began to be considered in medical literature. OERTEL (Jena 1733) discussed the delirious and demented cases, the 'furiosi' and 'menti capte'. The excited patient may injure himself or others. The demented lack judgment and commit stupid and unreasonable acts, including those which are caused by delusions. He offered good psychopathological examples to illustrate acute and chronic states. The problem of simulation of a psychosis was reviewed by GRAEBNER (Halle 1743). Other dissertations deal with legal aspects but do not offer sufficient psychopathological information. A third group was written from a judicial or theological point of view. Legal medicine began to be taught at the medical schools at the turn of the 18th century. In the second half of the century psychiatric dissertations in legal medicine were presented at the German medical schools and in the 19th century psychiatrists became actively interested, fully recognizing their obligation to the individual patient and to society.

Chapter X
Psychiatry and Social-Cultural Changes

The period from the 16th to the middle of the 18th century was one of rapid growth in medical knowledge and education. Current observations and a critical questioning of the past, as well as of new knowledge, replaced dogmatism in medicine. The clinical observations which were published in the 16th century were carefully reviewed and referred to in the textbooks of that period. They contained psychiatric case material which included description of symptoms, permitting a diagnosis and better formulation of the illness. Instead of a mere statement of the disease and an enumeration of time-honored symptoms the individual case was described. Increasingly the course of the illness was reviewed and evaluated in reaching a diagnosis. Psychology which was part of philosophy received critical attention, especially theological theories and mystical explanations which had been applied to the interpretations of clinical observations. Early dissertations attempted to evaluate these concepts. They added increasingly to WEYER's observations and statements, not only supporting but enlarging them.

Under the influence of DESCARTES' teaching, the relationship of body and mind and the influence of emotions were considered. A psychologically dynamic attitude became noticeable with the publication of WILLIS'[1] and later STAHL's psychological formulations[2]. The general treatment, based on humoral pathology, changed little. There was, however, a gradual development of psychotherapy.

During the 16th and 17th centuries religious unrest and intolerance and superstitions flourished. The individual was confronted by unanswerable questions. It is, therefore, not surprising that demonology continued to exert a strong influence even in the universities. The medical faculty at Halle was asked as late as 1723 for an opinion on the question of being possessed by the devil. FRIEDRICH HOFFMANN, an excellent

1   WILLIS, *op. cit.*
2   STAHL, *op. cit.*

diagnostician, wrote the opinion (*Medicina consultatoria 1724,* Decadis seconda, casus X). In his teaching and publications he had maintained a belief in the existence of the devil's powers. In discussing the case he was careful to be guided by medical facts. The patient was a 21-year-old farm-hand who insisted that he had made a pact with the devil and described this deed in detail, corresponding to the superstitious beliefs of the time. The opinion of the faculty was that attempts at seducing a person by the devil must be accepted. In this case, however, one had to consider the lack of good intelligence and education, a severe head injury at 13, the heavy drinking of brandy for several years, and the state of marked fear at the time of the examinations. The medical conclusion was that the statements were delusional.

In many universities the existence of demonology was discussed affirmitively by members of the faculties of medicine, philosophy and law[3]. In Wittenberg the topic appeared in several medical dissertations when TANDLER and SENNERT were the leading physicians of the faculty. These teachers as well as some in other medical schools felt it was the obligation of medicine to study current superstitious beliefs and their psychopathological meaning. The influence of fear, ecstatic experiences and delusions and later, suggestion, were considered. SENNERT's distinction between natural and diabolical lycanthropy was widely accepted[4]. Natural lycanthropy was a patient's delusion that he was a wolf. When bystanders believed that they saw the patient changed into a wolf, diabolical influences deluded their imagination. In the culturally advanced Strasbourg, FABRICIUS (1649) accepted this formulation. Much later, this psychopathological phenomenon was related to suggestion and still later called induced insanity.

In isolated parts of various countries, folklore and superstitions were prevalent for a long time after they had been rejected in the culturally advanced cities. One should consider this factor when one tries to evaluate statements in dissertations from universities such as Jena and Erfurt situated in small provincial towns, with many students coming from the wooded and mountainous surroundings.

The influence of the scientist, ROBERT BOYLE (1626–1691)[5], and later of the Leipzig professor of law, CHRISTIAN THOMASIUS

---

3   THORNDYKE, *op. cit.,* vol. VI and VII.
4   SENNERT, *op. cit.,* lib. II, part. III, sect. I, cap. VII.
5   BOYLE used SENNERT's statement of incantations to illustrate the uncritical attitude of physicians.

(1655–1728)[6], can be recognized in dissertations attacking superstition and witchcraft[7].

In the teaching of clinical medicine the various psychiatric disorders, including hysteria and hypochondriasis, were stressed. This fact becomes obvious from the publications of professors in their textbooks, observations and consultations, comments to dissertations and the journals of natural sciences[8]. Dissertations frequently offered a more detailed description of the psychological approach to patients than is found in textbooks[9].

6   CHRISTIAN THOMASIUS, teaching in Leipzig and Halle was the successful legal leader in the attack against superstition. To reach the legal group as well as the general public he wrote in Latin and German, including his influential small book *Von dem Laster der Zauberey*, 1706.

7   It is difficult to obtain a good understanding of living in the cities, small town and the countryside in the middle ages, the Renaissance and the 17th century. HAESER, *op. cit.*, stressed the importance of changes in dressing, living quarters and food, the prevailing powerty, the limitations forced by life in walled-in cities during the Renaissance and the 17th century. General health conditions in the western countries of Europe were reviewed by ROSEN, *op. cit.* SEBASTIAN FRANEK's *Germania Chronicon*, 1539 gives glimpses of life in German countries. Sculptures in French cathedrals and illuminated miniatures offer some information of life during the medieval period (J. Huizinga, *The Waning of the Middle Ages*, New York 1929). Paintings from 15th century Burgundy and the Flemish and German schools of the 16th and later centuries, confirm in detail the condensed statements which can be found in general literature of these periods. The books of FREYTAG, *op. cit.*, contain valuable lengthy excerpts from publications of the 16th to the 19th centuries.

H. RASHDALL *(op. cit.)* gives an understanding of life at the universities of the middle ages, FELIX PLATTER, *op. cit.* (autobiography), at the university of Montpellier and BAUER, *op. cit.*, and FREYTAG, *op. cit.*, at the German universities.

8   With the publications of medical journals, *Observationes and consultationes* ceased to be printed (18th century). Medical journals included brief psychiatric observations. At the beginning of the 19th century psychiatric periodicals appeared. Textbooks and treatises became influential in the 18th century.

9   Dissertations did not deal with idiocy and imbecillity except in brief references. The Greek an Latin writers included them under the term moria or stultitia. PLATTER, *op. cit.*, grouped these patients under hebetudo (idiocy), tarditas (imbecillity) and imprudentia (debility). He separated from them silliness (fatuitas) and childish behavior (infantia). Idiocy included cretinism which had already been noted by PARACELSUS. In the early 19th century cretinism was recognized as a thyroid disorder and well described psychiatrically. Educational efforts were directed at aiding them as well as other types of idiots and imbeciles. A hundred years later iodine deficiency was established as a cause for cretinism and the cause eliminated, resulting in the disappearance of the previously widespread cretinism. At

The progress in clinical psychiatry, as is demonstrated by many dissertations, is greater than has been assumed in historical psychiatric literature. Excitements were no longer considered an entity (mania) but separated into several groups which included our current manic, schizophrenic, epileptic and sexual excitements. It was recognized that melancholia covered various types of depression and schizophrenic illnesses. Post-partum psychoses were described. Catatonic stupor became separated from ecstatic conditions. The wide range of hysterical reactions became related and hypochondriacal symptoms better defined. Studying the course of the illness did not develop yet, but indications for such a need appear in several dissertations. There was a groping for the discovery of a clinical entity of excitement and depression. The concept of deterioration after excitement and in melancholia begins to be discussed. Post-mortem studies attracted increasing attention although the results were usually negative. Psychopathological descriptions became more detailed than previously and permitted a better understanding of delusions, visual hallucinations and the effects of anxiety and fear. The individual personality was considered and life situations were evaluated. The psychotic patient was recognized as a suffering person who needed sympathy and help.

In the second half of the 18th century progress continued at a more rapid pace, supported by the philosophies of the enlightment and the expansion of medical education. Publications, including dissertations, supported the development of psychiatry as a specialty.

It is difficult to compare disease pictures of different cultures. With environmental changes, including therapeutic and cultural influences, some psychopathological symptoms may become less frequent, others have varied their character, while a third group has become more obvious[10].

Diseases related to malnutrition and infections were important from the Renaissance to the 18th century. The corresponding psychiatric disorders were caused by damage to the brain and resulted in delirious reactions and psychoses related to inanition. Every physician was confronted by them and their descriptions can be found in the textbook the end of the 18th century schizophrenic dementia and later general paresis were separated from congenital and acquired dementia and in the present century further clarification has been obtained in this previously uniform group.

10   G. ROSEN discussed psychiatric illnesses in *Social attitudes to irrationality and madness,* J. H. Med. 1963, XVIII and *The mentally ill and the community,* J. H. Med. 1964, XIX.

since the time of HIPPOCRATES. The symptoms have not changed except for the hallucinations.

Infectious illnesses and their relationship to psychoses has, at different times, received considerable attention. PARÉ's[11] descriptions of the 16th century, based on his wide experience of wound infections, added more details but nothing fundamentally different. The same pertains to the frequent discussions in dissertations or to REIL's 18th century observations[12]. In the 20th century retentive memory disorders and amnesic disorders were stressed but these observations have been indicated in previous studies of delirium, especially those with resulting permanent brain damage.

Toxic deliria from drugs (cannabis indica, atropa belladonna, datura stramonium and hyoscyamus) have been mentioned frequently since the Renaissance. Some authors stressed vivid visual and tactile hallucinations which are not different from toxic reactions observed in drug addition of the last and present centuries. In the Renaissance some 'witches' experienced participation in sexual orgies with the devil and other participants. In the 20th century, sexual orgies with members of the participating group or with absent persons were hallucinated[13].

The marked decrease of delirious reactions in the last twenty years is related to generally improved health, to better physiological guidance in medical and surgical treatment and the control of infections by antibiotic drugs. The decrease of frequency of delirium tremens is unclear and its changing psychopathology. It is likely that dietary factors play a role. Delirium tremens was already described by HORST in 1628[14] but is rearely mentioned in medical literature before SUTTON's treatise (1813)[15]. In the succeeding years several publications from different countries appeared. There was no differentiation from other alcoholic psychoses to which probably the description of HIPPOCRATES and other early authors belong. The behavior in acute alcoholic intoxication has always been influenced by cultural attitudes, and the symptoms have

11   PARÉ, op. cit., gives a vivid picture of superstitions in the 16th century. He and FR. HOFFMANN in the 18th century demonstrate the mixture of a critical attitude in their observations and clinical interpretations and a lack of it to beliefs which could not be investigated.

12   JOHANN CHRISTIAN REIL, Über die Erkenntnis und Cur der Fieber.

13   H. W. MAIER, Der Kokainismus, Leipzig 1926.

14   GREGOR HORST, op. cit., lib. II, obs. XII and W. ROLFINCK, op. cit., lib. II, cons. IV.

15   F. THOMAS SUTTON, On delirium tremens, London 1813.

varied accordingly. For illustration one might consider the changes which have occurred in the 20th century. The acting out of a neurotic or psychopathic personality and the uncontrolled behavior which led to brawls and loss of human dignity is less marked. The factors affecting this change may be related to different toxic factors in the alcoholic beverages, to nutrition, and above all to cultural attitudes. Similar changes can be observed in drug addiction in different hospitals or cultural settings. Patients may react with mild or marked withdrawal symptoms to the same drugs and markedly different degrees of toxic excitements and hallucinations.

In this century changes in diet and in general hygiene have affected the clinical picture of deteriorating schizophrenia. Other symptoms which were considered important and frequently noted are now rarely seen. Catatonic symptoms, for instance, which thirty years ago were familiar to every medical student, now may not be seen by a psychiatrist during his entire three years of training. Catatonic posturing, including catalepsy and prolonged stupor are rarely encountered in a good psychiatric hospital where understanding and sympathy have replaced a domineering attitude. These symptoms had attracted and bewildered physicians since the 16th century. Echolalia, neologisms and mannerisms have become rare. The change seems to be related to a change in psychological attitude in the patient and his environment but may be also related to dietary and other factors which may have contributed to disorders of thinking and affected his psychological resistance. Symptoms have changed but the catatonic group can still be recognized. Insufficient control of bowels and bladder and the smearing of feces, described in early dissertations are no longer as important as twenty years ago. Destructiveness may occur in an outburst of anger which may be prevented by early recognition of the intense emotional reaction. Drugs which decrease anxiety, fear and resentment control many of these symptoms. Autistic withdrawal is noticeable in the activities of a group but not to the extreme and frequency as a few years ago when patients were permitted to lead isolated existences or when PLATTER kept them locked up in cells[16]. Considering the influence of cultural changes on the disappearance of schizophrenic symptoms, one must evaluate the ob-

16   F. PLATTER, observations, *op. cit.* The effect of the hospital environment on schizophrenic symptomatology during the last 150 years has not been sufficiently studied nor the effect of living in crowded cities, on isolated farms or in small villages.

servations that catatonic and marked autistic withdrawal reactions occur relatively frequently in primitive societies and in groups with inferior education or who feel oppressed. It has been demonstrated in clinical experience that the inability of communicating with schizophrenic patients and they with persons in their environment, much discussed in medical literature of the 19th and 20th centuries, is far less involved than was assumed. Isolation, fear, awe, ridicule, and rejection of others or by them are the dynamic forces which cause many schizophrenic symptoms.

The symptoms of ecstasy which are found in schizophrenia, epilepsy, manic excitements, brain disease, toxic influence and hysteria are more frequently observed in religious furor, in periods of cultural insecurities or in times when ecstasy is expected. It is a symptom which still occurs more readily in primitive people and in unintelligent and superstitious persons.

Until a few years ago involutional melancholia, with a well-defined group of symptoms, was widely accepted. This psychiatric picture has now practically disappeared, partly because treatment by electrically-induced convulsions can terminate this type of disorder early. In addition, however, some of the classical symptoms such as agitation, distorted hypochondriacal delusions, or delusions of excessive sinning, all of them mentioned in the medical literature of the last four hundred years, have become infrequent. At present they are occasionally observed in rural and non-sophisticated groups, but rarely in the educated and urban population. The changed attitude to menopause and to aging, as well as the better-preserved health and strength of this age group, have improved mental health and affected the psychopathologic picture. Depressive illnesses still occur to the problems of aging and attending insecurities and threats but the symptoms have changed.

An interesting example is presented by general paresis which was not described until the beginning of the 19th century[17]. Cases are found in the literature of the 17th century which might have been general paresis. With the decrease of syphilitic infections, and their early treatment, the illness has become less frequent. Successful treatment by malaria or penicillin has led to the early arrest of the illness or to recovery.

17 MÖNKEMÜLLER, *Zur Geschichte der progressiven Paralyse,* Neurol. Psych. 5: 500 (1911), after a careful review of the literature concluded that the increase of general paresis and the change in the clinical picture, expressed in psychopathologic and neurologic symptoms seemed to be related to the increasing stress and spread of civilization.

Some of these successfully treated patients, however, react with a schizophrenic, especially paranoid, psychopathologic picture. It is often impossible to distinguish these reactions from a true schizophrenic illness, when one sees these patients several years later. The grandiose psychopathologic behavior of general paresis, which was well-known in textbooks, became rare forty years ago, i.e., before modern treatment was available. The causes for this change have never been explained.

The relationship of depression and manic excitement has been mentioned in textbooks and dissertations. The few satisfactorily described cases correspond to those of modern times.

In medieval times and until the 18th century, hysterical symptoms were frequently related to religious aspects and to witchcraft. Somnambulic states, hysterical convulsions and opisthotonus seemed of utmost importance to the physicians. In the dissertations of the 17th and early 18th centuries somnambulic states and opisthotonus were less stressed. These dramatic and attention-getting symptoms reappeared at the end of the 18th century as a result of the widely advertised result by MESMER[18]; also, in the second half of the 19th century under the influence of CHARCOT's demonstrations[19]. In recent years the outstanding symptoms are phobias; varied physical symptoms which correspond to current illnesses, and sexual difficulties have taken their place. A considerable number of psychosomatic disorders and of anxiety symptoms may belong in this group.

In the 17th century the number of pilgrims and other wandering persons, including students, increased to such an extent that they became a problem of public health[20]. No psychiatric studies of the problem of vagabonds were made until the end of the 19th century. Among them are found a large number of schizophrenics, severe psychoneurot-

18 FRANZ ANTON MESMER, Mémoire sur la découverte du magnétisme animal, 1779. This book was followed by a large number of publications by himself and his enthusiastic disciples.

19 Like MESMER, the neurologist J. M. CHARCOT (1825–93) attracted great public acclaim by his dramatic clinic presentations of hypnotic opisthotonus and somnanbulism.

20 JUAN VIVES, De subventione pauperum, Bruges 1525, demanded that the government be responsible for the health of the poor and of the mentally ill. He urged to include also those from other countries who became sick. This group included pilgrims, students and vagabonds. His advice was followed in France, Germany and Spain. (During his reign, Philippe II kept an active interest in this problem which was especially troublesome in Spain with its large transient population.)

ics and psychopathic personalities[21]. There seems to be little doubt that those patients formed a considerable number of those with whom the Spanish and German authorities became concerned.

The hallucinations which have been most frequently mentioned since the late medieval centuries are visions of ghosts. With decreasing superstitious beliefs they became rare but they still occur in unintelligent persons from superstitious environments and in primitive people. They may be part of a schizophrenic illness, of depressed states with marked fear, of a senile reaction, of a delirium and of a hysterical reaction, especially in immature or unintelligent adolescents and children. Auditory hallucinations were described as thunder, trumpets and music, while voices are troubling the patients of our century. Tactile hallucinations of various types occurred in the past and now under the influence of fear, marked sexual excitement or toxic factors.

Many of these symptoms are increased or decreased by the belief and attitude of the physician. Examples are found in the attacks on witchcraft or its defense by physicians in the 16th and 17th centuries, in the discussion on tarantism in the 18th century and in the study and practice of hypnosis at the end of the 18th and 19th centuries.

Periods of war and famine do not affect mental health as strongly as that of emotional insecurity. Depressions and suicide increase little with persecutions and external danger but much with loneliness and doubts in the worthwhileness of living. These conclusions are supported by the suicidal wave in young educated people in England and France of the 18th century[22]. Support by the group permits the individual to suffer and tolerate the aggression from the environment, as seen in the period of persecutions from the 14th through the 16th centuries and in the 20th century. In some persons it is religious and philosophic beliefs which give strength, in others suggestion[23].

21   KARL WILMANNS, *Zur Psychopathologie des Landstreichers,* Leipzig 1906.
22   MOREAU (DE TOURS) fils, *De la contagion du suicide,* Paris, 1875; ALEXANDRE BRIERRE DE BOISMONT, *Du suicide et de la folie suicide, considérés dans leur rapports avec la statistique, la médicine et la philosophie,* Paris 1856.
23   The strengthening of mental health and the prevention of psychiatric disorders has been treated in medical literature by several authors who had considerable influence in medicine. Their discussions reveal their personal attitude and the period in which they lived: MARSILIUS FICINUS, *De vita libri tres,* Basel 1549, represents the early Renaissance; GREGOR HORST, *De tuenda sanitate studiosorum et litteratorum,* Marburg 1628, the late German humanist period; JEROME GAUB, *De regimine mentis,* Leyden 1747 and 1763, the scientific period of Holland; JOHANN

The suggestive influence of fear and its infectious nature has troubled physicians and governments during an acute phase of plague (13th and 14th centuries) and was observed in the panics which involved the civilian population and soldiers in the wars of the 20th century.

The 16th century has been called the century of suggestion; the present, that of anxiety. Psychopathological symptoms will be affected differently but there are no indications of new psychiatric illnesses under different conditions.

C. A. HEINROTH, *Der Schlüssel zu Himmel und Hölle im Menschen, oder über moralische Kraft und Passivität,* Leipzig 1829, the early Romantic period of Northern Germany and ERNST VON FEUCHTERSLEBEN, *Zur Diätetik der Seele,* Wien 1838, the end of the romantic period in Vienna.

Bibliography

I. Observationes (including Consultationes and Epistolae)

1 AMATUS LUSITANUS: Curationum medicinalium centuriae septem. Venice 1557.

2 BALLONIUS (BAILLOU, DE), GUILIELMUS: Consiliorum medicinalium liber I. Paris 1635.

3 BENEVIENI, ANTONIO: De abditis nonnullis ac mirandis morborum et sanationum causis; in GATINARIA, MARCUS, Contenta in hoc volumine sunt infra notata. Venice 1516.

4 FABRICIUS HILDANUS, GUILIELMUS: Opera omnia. Frankfurt 1682.

5 FERNEL, JEAN: Universa medicina. Genève 1680.

6 FORESTUS (FOREEST, VAN), PETRUS: Observationum et curationum medicinalium ac chirurgicarum opera omnia. Frankfurt 1634.

7 HEER, HENRICUS AB: Observationes medicae. Liège 1631.

8 HORSTIUS (HORST), GREGOR: Observationum medicinalium singularium libri V. Ulm 1625.

9 LANGIUS (LANGE), JOHANNES: Epistolarum medicinalium libri III. Frankfurt 1589.

10 LOMMIUS (LOMM, VAN), JODOCUS: Observationum medicinalium. Amsterdam 1715.

11 MERCURIALIS, HIERONYMUS: Liber responsorium et consultationum medicinalium. Basel 1588.

12 MONTANUS (MONTE), GIOVANNI BATTISTA: Consultationes medicae. Antea quidum Ioannis Cratonis opera atque studio. Basel 1572.

13 PLATER (PLATTER), FELIX: Observationum ... Libre tres. Basel 1641. Histories and Observations upon most Diseases. (Transl. by COLE and CULPEPER.) London 1664.

14 RIVERIUS (RIVIÈRE), LAZARUS: Opera medica universa. Frankfurt 1669.

15 ROLFINCIUS (ROLFINCK), GUERNERIUS: ... Ordo et methodus medicinae specialis consultatoriae ... continens consilia medica, ad normam veterum et novorum dogmatum adornata. Jena 1669.

16 RULAND, MARTIN: Curationum epyricarum et historicarum, centuriae decem. Leyden 1628.

17 SALMUTH, PHILIP: Observationum medicarum centuriae tres. Brunswick 1648.

18 SCHENCK, JOHANN: Observationae medicae rarae. Frankfurt 1665.

19 SOLENANDER, REINERT: Consilorium medicinalium sectiones V. Frankfurt
    1596.
20 TULPIUS (TULP), NIC.: Observationes medicae. Amsterdam 1672.
21 VALLERIOLA, FRANCISCUS: Observationum medicinalium libri sex. Lyon 1573.
22 WEPFER, JOHANN JACOB: Observationes medico-practicae. Schaffhausen 1727.
23 ZACUTUS LUSITANUS, ABRAHAM: De medicorum principum historia libri VI.
    Leyden 1642.

II. Textbooks

1   AVICENNA: Canon medicinae. Venice 1595.
2   BOERHAAVE, HERMANN: Aphorisimi de cognoscendis et curandis morbis. Ley-
    den 1737.
3   DIEMERBROECK, ISBRANDUS DE: ... Opera omnia, anatomica et medica. Utrecht
    1685.
4   ETTMÜLLER, MICHAEL: Opera omnia theoretica et practica. Leyden 1685.
5   FERNEL, JEAN: Universa medicina. Genève 1680.
6   FONTANONUS, DYONISIUS: De morborum internorum curatione. Lyon 1549.
7   FRACASTORIUS, HIERONYMUS: Opera omnia. Venice 1584.
8   GATINARIA, MARCUS: De curis egretudinum particularium novi Almansoris
    Practica. Venice 1521.
9   GUAINERIO, ANTONIO: Practica. Lyon 1517.
10 LAURENTIUS (DU LAURENS), ANDR.: Opera omnia anatomica et medica. Frank-
    furt 1627.
11 PISO, NICOLAUS: De cognoscendis et curandis praecipue internis humani cor-
    poris morbis libri tres ... Frankfurt 1585.
12 PLATER (PLATTER), FELIX: Praxeos medicae opus. Basel 1666. A Golden Prac-
    tice of Physick. (Transl. by COLE and CULPEPER.) London 1662.
13 RHAZES: ... Tractatus nonus ad Regem Almansorem. De curatione morborum
    particularium; opusculum huic faeculo accommodatissimum. Paris 1534.
14 RIVERIUS (RIVIÈRE), LAZARUS: Opera medica universa. Frankfurt 1669.
15 RONDELETUS (RONDELET), GUILIELMUS: Methodus curandorum omnium mor-
    borum corporis humani in tres libros distincta. Paris 1574.
16 SAXONIA, HERCULES: Opera practica. Padua 1639.
17 SENNERT, DANIEL: Institutionum medicinae libri V. Wittenberg 1628. Practi-
    cae medicinae liber primus. Wittenberg 1636.
18 SYDENHAM, THOMAS: Praxis medica s. opuscula universa. Leipzig 1695. Praxis
    medica. The Practice of Physick. (Transl. by WILLIAM SALMON.) London
    1716.
19 WILLIS, THOMAS: Opera omnia. Genève 1579. Two Discourses concerning the
    Soul of Brutes. (Transl. of De anima brutorum, by S. PORDAGE.) London
    1683.
20 ZACCHIAS, PAUL: Quaestionum medico-legalium tomus primus, secundus, ter-
    tius. Lyon 1701.

III. General Literature

1 BAUER, MAX: Sittengeschichte des deutschen Studententums. Dresden 196 . .
2 AFNAN, SOHEIL M.: Avicenna, His Life and Works. London 1958.
3 BARON, HYACINTHE THEODORE: Quaestionum medicarum series chronologica (1539–1752). Paris 1752.
4 BAUER, MAX: Sittengeschichte des deutschen Studententums. Dresden 196 . .
5 BECKER, W. M.: Die Universität Giessen von 1607 bis 1907. Giessen 1907.
6 BINZ, CARL: Doctor Johann Weyer, ein rheinischer Arzt, der erste Bekämpfer des Hexenwahns. Berlin 1896.
7 BOERHAAVE, HERMAN: SWIETEN, GERARD VAN – The Commentaries upon the Aphorisms of HERMAN BOERHAAVE ... (Transl. into English.) London 1744–1773.
8 BOOS, HEINRICH: PLATTER, THOMAS and FELIX – Zur Sittengeschichte des 16. Jahrhunderts. Leipzig 1878.
9 BURCKHARDT, A.: Geschichte der Medizinischen Fakultät zu Basel, 1466–1900. Basel 1917.
10 CAELIUS AURELIANUS: On Acute Diseases and On Chronic Diseases. Ed. and transl. by I. E. DRABKIN. Chicago 1950.
11 CALMEIL, L. F.: De la Folie considérée sous le point de vue pathologique, philosophique, historique et judiciaire depuis la Renaissance des Sciences en Europe jusqu'à 19e Siècle. Paris 1845.
12 CASTELLI (CASTELLUS), BARTHOLOMAEUS: Lexicum medicum, novae ed. JOANNIS RHODII. Leyden 1721.
13 CASTIGLIONI, ARTURO: A History of Medicine. (Transl. from the Italian and ed. by E. B. KRUMBHAAR.) New York 1941.
14 DELAUNAY, P.: La Vie Médicale. Paris 1935.
15 DIEPGEN, PAUL: Geschichte der Medizin; die historische Entwicklung der Heilkunde und des ärztlichen Lebens. Berlin 1953.
16 FALK, F.: Studien über Irrenheilkunde der Alten. Allg. Psychiat. *23:* 419 (1866).
17 FEHR, HANS: Massenkunst im 16. Jahrhundert. Berlin 1924.
18 FREYTAG, GUSTAV: Bilder aus der deutschen Vergangenheit. Leipzig 1895.
19 FRIEDENWALD, HARRY: The Jews and Medicine. Essays. Baltimore 1944.
20 FRIEDRICH, J. B.: Versuch einer Literärgeschichte der Pathologie und Therapie der Psychischen Krankheiten, von den ältesten Zeiten bis zum Neunzehnten Jahrhundert. Würzburg 1830.
21 GALEN, CLAUDIUS GALENI: Opera omnia. (Ed. C. G. KÜHN.) Leipzig 1821–1833. Oeuvres de Galien. Transl. CH. DAREMBERG. (Des lieux affectés, vol. III, chap. IX.) Paris 1854–1856.
22 GRANJEL, LUIS S.: Historia de la Medicina Española. Barcelona 1962.
23 GUARINONIUS, HIPPOLITUS: Die grewel der Verwüstung Menschlichen Geschlechts. Ingolstadt 1610.
24 HAESER, HEINRICH: Lehrbuch der Geschichte der Medizin und der epidemischen Krankheiten. Jena 1875–1882.
25 HALLER, ALBERT V.: Bibliotheca medicinae practicae. Basel and Bern 1788.

26 HECKER, J. F. C.: The Epidemics of the Middle Ages. (Transl. by B. G. BABINGTON.) London 1844.

27 HIGHMORE, NATHANAEL: De passione hysterica. Amsterdam 1660.

28 HIPPOCRATES: The genuine works of Hippocrates. (Transl. by F. ADAMS.) London 1849.

29 HIRSCH, A.: Geschichte der medizinischen Wissenschaften in Deutschland. München 1893.

30 HUIZINGA, J.: The Waning of the Middle Ages. New York 1924.

31 HUSNER, FRITZ: Verzeichnis der Basler medizinischen Universitätsschriften von 1575–1829. Basel 1942.

32 IRSAY, STEPHEN D': Histoire des Universités Françaises et Etrangères. Paris 1933.

33 ISLER, HANSRUEDI: THOMAS WILLIS – Ein Wegbereiter der modernen Medizin. Stuttgart 1965.

34 LAEHR, HEINRICH: Die Literatur der Psychiatrie, Neurologie und Psychologie von 1459–1799. Berlin 1900.

35 LAIGNEL-LAVASTINE et GUEGAN, B.: Histoire Générale de la Médecine. Paris 1936–1949.

36 LEGRAND, NOÉ: La Collection des Thèses de l'Ancienne Faculté de Médecine de Paris depuis 1539 et son Catalogue inédit jusqu'en 1793. Paris 1914.

37 LEMNIUS, LEVINUS: De miraculis occultis naturae libri III. Frankfurt 1628.

38 MEIBOMIUS, JOHN HENRY: A Treatise on the Use of Flogging in Medicine and Venery. (Transl. from the Latin by a Physician.) Paris 1898.

39 MINDER, ROBERT: Der Hexenglaube bei den Iatrochemikern des 17. Jahrhunderts. Dissertation. Zürich 1963.

40 MORGENTHALER, WALTER: Bernisches Irrenwesen von den Anfängen bis zur Eröffnung des Tollhauses 1749. Bern 1915.

41 RASHDALL, HASTINGS: The Universities of Europe in the Middle Ages. London 1936.

42 RATHER, L. J.: Mind and Body in Eighteenth Century Medicine. A Study based on JEROME GAUB's De regimine mentis. Berkeley 1966.

43 RAYNAUD, MAURICE: Les Médecins au Temps de Molière. Paris 1863.

44 ROSEN, GEORGE: A History of Public Health. New York 1958.

45 SCHIPPERGES, HEINRICH: Ideologie und Historiographie des Arabismus. Sudhoffs Archiv für Geschichte der Medizin und der Naturwissenschaften. Beiheft I (1961).

46 SHERRINGTON, CHARLES: The Endeavour of Jean Fernel. CAMBRIDGE 1946.

47 SPRENGEL, KURT: Versuch einer Pragmatischen Geschichte der Arzneykunde. Halle 1821.

48 STAHL, GEORG ERNST: Theoria medica vera. Halle 1708. Über den mannigfaltigen Einfluss von Gemütsbewegungen auf den menschlichen Körper. (Transl. BERNWARD, JOSEF GOTTLIEB.) Leipzig 1961.

49 SYDENHAM, THOMAS: De affectione hysterica. Dissertatio epistolaris ad GUILIEMUS COLE, M. D. London 1682.

50 TEMKIN, OWSEI: The Falling Sickness. Baltimore 1945.

51 THORNDYKE, LYNN: A History of Magic and Experimental Science. New York 1958.
52 TREND, J. B.: The Civilization of Spain. London 1963.
53 VEITH, ILZA: Hysteria. The History of Disease. Chicago 1965.
54 WIERUS (WEYER), JOHANN: Opera omnia. Amsterdam 1660.
55 ZILBOORG, GREGORY: A History of Medical Psychology. By GREGORY ZIL-BOORG in collaboration with GEORGE W. HENRY. New York 1941.

Appendix
List of Dissertations

The correct term for a dissertation was 'dissertatio inauguralis', inauguralis indicating the ceremonial installation to the office. In many universities different terms were printed; e.g. 'disputatio inauguralis', 'quaestio', 'animadversiones', 'positiones'. These dissertations or disputations for the degree *(pro gradu)* form the largest part of this list but included are also disputations which were required at stated intervals ('exercitii gratia'). They are frequently recognized by having more than one respondent on the title page.

The printing of dissertations started in the latter part of the 16th century and was requested in Basel in 1575, and during the end of the 16th and the beginning of the 17th centuries by most other universities. Italian universities did not request the printing of dissertations until the 18th century. Their influence on medical literature was, therefore, negligible.

Dissertations were printed in small editions (probably 200–300 copies), loosely bound and usually without a cover. Thus, they became easily lost. Wars and incidental fires destroyed many libraries, especially in this century. Many universities were careless in keeping lists of the names of students and their publications. In Paris, under dean Hy-ACINTHE THEODORE BARON († 1758) and his son, who succeeded him, the manuscript of every thesis since the 16th century was printed in one copy (1752). Another complete collection of dissertations is found at Basel; a list of all dissertations of Holland is available at the library of the University of Amsterdam.

The year on printed dissertations may not be the accurate date of the promotion because they may have been reprinted later. As a rule, the printers of dissertations were assigned by the universities where the degree was obtained. Sometimes the reprints were made by a printer in the student's home town, or in another university town, to which the author had moved.

Dissertations and theses were printed in quarto; their length, in addition to the title page, varies from 4 to 20 pages or longer. Many German dissertations contain several pages of dedication, e.g. to a prince or a famous person, and of laudatory remarks by the professor and friends, frequently in the form of poems. The dissertations were written in Latin, but some of the poems were in German.

Some of the dissertations have a preface *(proempticon),* written by a professor, who may have been, but was not necessarily, the presiding professor. These prefaces are frequently very informative. They offer the professor an opportunity to express himself on a topic which may not relate directly to the content of the dissertation.

After the conclusion of the dissertation, the student may add a *corollaria* in which he makes several brief statements which were too tangential to be included in the dissertation. In the succeeding chapters there are references to *corollaria* and *encomiums.*

The title page contains the full title of the dissertation, the university, the presiding professor, the dean or rector, the respondent (student), his place of birth, the date and place of printing. There are many dissertations in which some of this data is omitted. The information which is always contained is the title, the respondent, and the date and place of printing. In most German universities the dean and professor is mentioned. In Basel less than 30 percent of the names of the presiding professors appear. In the dissertations of Edinburgh and Holland the professor's name is rarely given, but always that of the rector of the university. In Paris all the professors of the faculty signed the thesis, with the presiding officer designated as such. In Montpellier, the professor signed in a presiding or promoting capacity.

The title page may be simple, or very elaborate, apparently depending on the taste and financial means of the student or his backer. In Holland, the seal of the university occupies an important place.

The humanistic custom of authors selecting a Greek name, or coining a new name, does not enter this review. The only exception is ERASTUS, Professor of Medicine in Basel and Heidelberg, whose name is THOMAS LIEBLER. More troublesome to the modern reader is the humanistic tendency to translate a German name into its Latin equivalent. Whenever possible, the German name is used in this monograph and, if indicated, the Latin form is in parenthesis.

Latin names which have become accepted in modern historical books, e.g. CAMERARIUS, are given in this form as the actual German name would add confusion.

The Latinizing of a name by adding 'us' or 'ius' is easily recognized. It should, however, be kept in mind that double consonants were not used in Latin, e.g., PLATTER appears as PLATER. In French or Dutch names, the modern usage of publications is applied throughout and shown in parenthesis may be the name as it appeared on the title page.

The names of the students (respondents) are listed alphabetically. When they could not be established, the dissertations are listed under the name of the presiding professor. In such a case the name listed is put in parenthesis. When original dissertations could not be located, possible misspelling was unavoidable.

At the beginning of the 19th century the Prussian educational authorities decided to list dissertations under the professor's name as author, a system accepted finally by all the German libraries. This policy may make it difficult to find a certain publication because perhaps in a reference in a book or in another dissertation the student's name was mentioned as the author. Some professors had a collection of dissertations, which were written under their guidance, printed in one volume. The names of the students may or may not be mentioned. In rare cases a professor may actually have printed a group of dissertations as if they were separate chapters of a book.

The role of the professor is disputable. His name may appear because he was really a co-author, to satisfy his need for recognition, because he wanted to share the responsibility with the neophyte, or to enable the student to attain special recognition from the sponsor's academic reputation. There is no general conclusion and each dissertation has to be evaluated. In Reims some professors had printed 'auctor' behind their names, indicating that the professor and not the respondent had written the dissertation. In German universities 'auctor' appears occasionally behind the respondent's name.

A professor may give in the same year the same topic to two different students. The first dissertation was then called 'disputatio prior', the second 'disputatio posterior'. Printed disputations may also include two respondents who discussed two different aspects of the question submitted to them.

In the 16th century, in the examination for the doctoral degree, the student was asked to comment on a passage from the books of HIPPO-CRATES or GALEN. In the 17th century, the professor might offer a lengthy discussion of a topic and put specific questions to the students. The printed answer took sometimes the place of a dissertation.

Dissertations

The dissertations are listed under the name of the student (respondent). When the name could not be established the professor's name is given (in parenthesis). The numbers in parenthesis indicate university and other libraries where copies are available, a small 'a' that the dissertation was reprinted in the professors collected works:

Basel (1)
Bethesda, Md, National Library of Medicine (2)
Cracow, Jagiellonion Library (3)
Erlangen (4)
Göttingen (5)
Jena (6)
Leipzig (7)
Leyden (8)
London, British Museum (9)
London, Welcome Historical Medical Library (10)
Montpellier (11)
München (12)
New York, Payne Whitney Psychiatric Clinic, Cornell University (13)
Paris, Bibliothèque de la Faculté de Médecine (14)
Reims (15)
Strasbourg (16)
Tübingen (17)
Utrecht (18)
Wien, Institut für Geschichte der Medizin (19)
Zürich, Zentralbibliothek (20)
Copenhagen (21)
Giessen (22)
Groningen (23)
Rostock (24)

Library

1 ABRAHAM, HEINRICH – Prof. TOBIAS TANDLER: De fascino et incantatione. Wittenberg 1605 (13a).
2 ABRAHAMOWITZ, MEYER – Prof. GRUNERT: De spirituosorum liquorum noxa atque utilitate. Halle 1743 (18).

3   ACOLUTHUS, JEAN – Prof. P. RAINSSANT (author): An narcotica aphrodiasiacis medicamentis miscenda? Reims 1680.

4   ACOLUTHUS, JO. C. – Prof. ABR. VATER: De sympatheticis curationibus medico rationali indignis et illicitis. Wittenberg 1723 (18).

5   ADRIANUS, MENSO: De affectione hypochondriaca. Utrecht 1704 (2, 9, 17).

6   AEMYLIUS, LEONHARD – Prof. JACKOB HORST: De memoriae deperditae curanda ratione in genere. Jena 1609 (9, 13a).

7   AESCHARDT, J.: De vi imaginationis. Jena 1598.

8   ALBECK, ERNEST JOSEPH – Prof. ELIAS RUDOLPH CAMERARIUS: Casus de agritudine animi. Tübingen 1688 (5, 10, 17).

9   ALBERTI, MICHAEL – Prof. GEORG ERNST STAHL: De hypochondriaco – Hysterico malo. Halle 1703 (2, 4, 5, 9) (see GRAEBNER).

10   (ALBERTI, MICHAEL): De melancholia vera et simulata. Halle 1743.

11   ALBINUS, BERNHARDUS: De catalepsi. Leyden 1676 (10, 13, 19).

12   ALBRECHT, OTTO GOTTFRIED – Prof. ANDREAS ELIAS BUECHNER: De morbis cerebri ex structura ejus anatomica deducendis. Erfurt 1741 (5).

13   AMERSFOORT, JACOBUS: De hysterica passione. Utrecht 1694 (17).

14   AMMAN, G. CHR. – Prof. WERNER ROLFINCK: De uteri suffocatione. Jena 1661 (13a).

15   ANDERSON, G. – Prof. BERNH. ALBINUS: De affectibus hypochondriacis. Leyden 1695.

16   ANDREA, ERDMANN FRIEDRICH – Prof. RUDOLF WILHELM CRAUSIUS: De passione hysterica strangulatoria. Jena 1710 (5).

17   ANDREAE, CHRISTIAN EBERHARD – Prof. ALEXANDER CAMERARIUS: Num mania sit apyretos. Tübingen 1734 (4, 9, 19, 20).

18   ANDRIESSEN, JACOBUS JOHANNES: De maternorum imaginationum et animi pathematum in foetum efficacia. Utrecht 1748 (17).

19   ANOMOEUS, JOHANNES JOACHIMUS – Prof. TOBIAS TANDLER: De melancholia indicationibus prognosticis et curatione. Wittenberg 1608 (13a).

20   AQUIN, ANDONIUS D': An chlorosi venus? Montpellier 1647 (11).

21   ARCELIN, P. – Prof. LUDOVICUS-PETRUS LE HOC: An aqua vitae aqua mortis? Paris 1743 (14).

22   (ARNISAEUS, HENNING): De melancholia hypochondriaca. Helmstadt 1620 (2).

23   ARNISAEUS, FRIDERICUS – Prof. OLAUS WORMIUS: De affectione melancholiae hypochondriacae. Copenhagen 1654 (2).

24   ARNOLDUS, JOHANNES PETRUS: De suffocatione hysterica. Utrecht 1701 (9).

25   AUGIER, ROB. – Prof. THOMAS ERASTUS: De animae facultatibus. Basel 1583 (1).

26   AYRER, CHRISTOPHORUS SEBASTIANUS – Prof. WERNER ROLFINCK: De phrenitide. Jena 1632 (4, 13a).

27   BACHGALLUS, MICHAEL – Prof. WERNER ROLFINCK: De mania. Jena 1633 (1, 9, 12, 13a, 16).

28   BACMEISTER, JOANNES – Prof. WILHELM LAUREN: Propositiones sequentes de melancholia. Rostock 1593 (9).

29   BACKHAUS, AUGUSTINUS SEVERUS – Prof. AUGUST HEINRICH FASCH: De amore insano. Jena 1686 (4, 5, 13, 17, 18).

30 BADTZMANN: De affectione hypochondriaca. Leiden 1643 (23).

31 BAGNOLS, JOSEPHUS: Morbos internos capitis et thoracis ad pathologiam referre. Montpellier 1710 (11).

32 BAJERUS, JOHANN JACOB – Prof. GEORG WOLFFGANG WEDEL: De amore. Jena 1698 (4).

33 (BAIER, JOHANN JACOB): De memoria. Altdorf 1708 (4).

34 BAIER, WILHELM – Prof. S. JAC. AURACHER: De memoria. Altdorf 1706.

35 BARADAT, ANTONIUS – Prof. JACQUES LAZERME: De somnambulatione. Montpellier 1748 (11).

36 BARCKHUYSEN, OTTO: Sistens considerationem terroris pathologico-therapeuticam. Leyden 1738 (8).

37 BARFEKNECHT, OTTO CASIM. – Prof. HIERON. COSNIER: An melancholicis balanem? Paris 1731 (4).

38 BARTH, JOH. CONRAD – Prof. JOH. RUD. SALZMANN: De phanthasiae actionibus in corpus. Strasbourg 1653.

39 BATTUS, CONR.: De melancholia hypochondriaca. Rostock 1605 (4, 24).

40 BATTUS, JACOBUS – Prof. JOHANN LEMBKEN: De spiritibus ardentibus per abusum, morborum causis, ejusdemque therapia – Oder von dem Brandtwein, und denen sogenannten Liqueures, auch deren Missbrauch als Ursachen vieler Kranckheiten des menschlichen Körpers und wie demselben abzuhelfen. Greifswald 1733 (2).

41 BAUSCH, LEONHARD: De vera phrenitide. Basel 1601 (1, 13).

42 BECK, HENRICUS JACOBUS: De ebrietate. Heidelberg 1746.

43 BECKHER, DANIEL: De affectu hypochondriaco. Königsberg 1623 (7).

44 BECKMANN, WILH.: De affectione hypochondriaca. Leyden 1676 (8, 9).

45 BEER, LEONHARD: De affectibus capitis internus. Leipzig 1657.

46 BEHNKEN – Prof. CASPAR POSNER: De memoriae adminiculis. Jena 1689.

47 BEHRENS, CONRAD BARTHOLD – Prof. HENRICUS MEIBOM: De suffocatione hysterica. Helmstadt 1684 (2, 4–6, 9).

48 BEHRENS, CAROLUS LUDWIG – Prof. MICHAEL ALBERTI: De solitudinis medica utilitate. Halle 1737 (13).

49 BEHRISCH, CHRISTIAN GOTTOFREDUS – Prof. MICHAEL ALBERTI: De phantasiae usu et abusu in medicina. Halle 1722 (4, 6, 9 10).

50 BELINUS A BELLFORT, ZACHAR: De melancholia. Basel 1607 (1, 13).

51 BELLANGER, FRANCISCUS ADOLPHUS: De animi pathematis. Leyden 1664 (8).

52 BELLETESTE, JOANNES JACOBUS – Prof. LUDOVICUS CLAUDIUS BOURDELIN: An hypochondriaci morbi remedium Equitatio? Paris 1737 (14).

53 BELOV, JAC. CHN. – Prof. ECCARD LEICHNER: De matrona hypochondriaca. Erfurt 1685 (5).

54 BEN, JOHANNES: De suffocatione hypochondriaca. Leyden 1683 (8).

55 BENDER, J. H. – Prof. HILCHEN: Triga observationum medicarum. Giessen 1748.

56 BENIER, PETRUS: De phrenitide. Leyden 1682 (1, 8, 17, 23).

57 BERARD, JOANN. STEPH.: De phrenitide vera. Leyden 1745 (8).

58 BERCHER, PETRUS – Prof. ACHILLE-FRANCISCO FONTAINE: An melancholicis peregrinatio? Paris 1741 (9).

59   BERCKE, JOHANN – Prof. GEORG CHRISTOPH. PETRI: Passionem hystericam. Erfurt 1672 (5).

60   BERG, GEORGIUS LEONHARDUS DE – Prof. JOANNES HENRICUS SCHULZE: De vino interdicendes. Halle 1735 (16).

61   BERGER, CLAUDIUS – Prof. ROBERT RAOULT: Est-ne imperfectus qui Astrologiam ignorat Medicus? Paris 1667 (9).

62   BERGER, CHRISTIAN GOTTLIEB: De melancholia hypochondriaca. Frankfurt a. O. 1715 (12).

63   (BERGER, JO. JUSTUS DE): De puerperarum mania et melancholia. Göttingen 1745 (9).

64   BERNARD, JOANNES STEPHANUS: De phrenitide vera. Leyden 1745 (1, 4, 8, 12).

65   BEUTTEL – Prof. GODOFREDUS MOEBIUS: De mania sive insania. Jena 1648.

66   BEX, ABRAHAM: De melancholia. Utrecht 1680.

67   BEYER, ANDRIAN – Prof. JOHANN HANKIUS: De ira. Jena 1653 (6).

68   BEYER, JOHANN HARTMANN – Prof. ANDREAS PLANER: De furore, seu mania; eiusque curatione. Tübingen 1588 (16, 20).

69   BEYERLEIN, JOH. CHRISTOPHORUS – Prof. LAURENTIUS THEOPHIL LUTHER: Sistens indolun et curam phrenitidis. Erfurt 1733 (2).

70   BEZEL, ANDREAS CHRISTIANUS – Prof. JOANNES HENRICUS SCHULZE: De paraphrenitide. Halle 1742 (2, 18).

71   BEZOLDUS, CASPARUS – Prof. RUDOLF WILHELM CRAUSIUS: De phrenitide. Jena 1689 (4, 5, 10).

72   BIARD, GABRIEL – Prof. CLAUDIUS BOYVIN: An melancholiae hypochondriacae tenos sectio? Paris 1608 (14).

73   BICQUET, ANSELMUS – Prof. JOANNE AKAKIA: An phrenitidi arteriotoma? Paris 1630 (14).

74   BIECK – Prof. CHRISTIAN ROCHRENSEE: De autocheirias. Wittenberg 1702.

75   BIELER, AMBROSIUS CAROLUS – Prof. CHRISTIAN LUDWIG WUCHERER: De amore insano. Jena 1717 (4, 5).

76   BIELITZ – Prof. LAURENTIUS HEISTER: De mania. Helmstadt 1725 (2).

77   BILGER, JOHANN – Prof. GREGOR HORST: De elementis ac temperamentis. Giessen 1609 (13a).

78   BILITZER, CHRISTOPHORUS – Prof. GREGOR HORST: De pulso amatoria. Giessen 1611 (13a).

79   BILSTEIN, JOHANN ULRICH – Prof. JUSTUS HENRICUS MANGOLDT: De delirio. Erfurt 1681 (4, 5, 12, 16, 17).

80   BING: De delirio febrili. Halle 1733.

81   BINGER, CASPAR – Prof. GREGOR HORST: De elementis ac temperamentis. Giessen 1609 (13a).

82   BLANC, ANDREAS: An catalepsi per periodos recurrenti pulvis kinae-kinae? Montpellier 1702 (11).

83   BLANCHARD, JEAN – Prof. THOMAS LE FRICQUE (author): An Venus salubris? Reims 1690 (15).

84   BLANQUET, SAMUEL: An venenum tarantulae scorpioni viperae et canis rabidi, primario spiritus inficiat? Montpellier 1711 (11).

85 BLEKER, GEORGIUS FRIDERICUS – Prof. CASPAR MARCHER: De melancholia hy-
     pochondriaca. Kiel 1673 (4, 5).

86 BLOCHMANN, JOHANNES GOTTLIEB – Prof. FRIEDRICH HOFFMANN: De morbis
     ex atonia cerebri nervorumque nascentibus. Halle 1708 (2, 6, 9).

87 BLOUET, LUC ABRAHAM – Prof. H. MARCQUART: An sanitati matrimonium?
     Reims 1704 (15).

88 BLUM, EMANUEL – Prof. MICHAEL ETTMÜLLER: De dolore hypochondriaco,
     vulgò fed falsò putato splenetico. Leipzig 1683 (13).

89 BLUM, MAURICIUS: De melancholia hypochondriaca. Wittenberg 1629.

90 BLUMBERG, GOTHOFREDO GUILIELMO – Prof. GEORG WOLFFGANG WEDEL: Ve-
     nus medica et morbofera. Jena 1685 (4).

91 BODAEUS, EGBERT – Prof. Jo. HEURNEUS: De phrenitide. Leyden 1597.

92 BOECKELER, J.: De ira. Strasbourg 1716.

93 BÖHMER: De iracundia. Helmstadt 1694.

94 BOHMER, MARTINUS FRIDERICUS – Prof. JOANNE JUNCKER: Casum Cuiusdam
     matronae largissimo opii usu per plures annos tractatae. Halle 1744.

95 BOEHMIUS, ANDREAS – Prof. ADOLPH HARTMANN: Exhibens statum furiosorum
     in paroxysmo constitutorum. Marburg 1740 (2).

96 BOERHAAVE, HERMANNUS: De distinctione mentis a corpore. Leyden 1690 (8).

97 BÖSCH, JOHANN WOLFFG. – Prof. CASPAR POSNER: Miscellanea de anima.
     Jena 1671.

98 BOIRE, ANDREAS: An catalepsi pulvis kinae-kinae? Montpellier 1706 (11).

99 BOLLMANN, JOH. HENRICH: De catalepsi. Marburg 1693 (5).

100 BOLSTER, JO. H. – Prof. G. E. HAMBERGER: De hypnoticis et narcoticis. Jena
     1748 (4).

101 BONETUS, JOACHIMUS: An uterinae suffocationi graveolentia? Montpellier
     1619 (11).

102 BONNE-MAISON, ALPH. DE – Prof. ANTON MATTHAEUS: De melancholia hypo-
     chondriaca. Leyden 1678 (8).

103 BÖNNEKEN, JOAN. WOLFGANG FRIDERICUS – Prof. D. PLACIDUS: Sistans me-
     lancholia vulgo. Die Schwermütigkeit. Erfurt 1728 (2, 17, 19).

104 BONVOUST, FRANCISCUS TIBERIUS: De phrenitide. Utrecht 1743 (18).

105 BORNEMANN, COSMUS: De melancholia. Basel 1594 (1).

106 BORREBAGH, HENRICUS – Prof. HERMANN WITSIUS: De melancholia. Utrecht
     1738 (18).

107 BOUCHETAL, ANDREAS – Prof. PETRUS LE PESCHEUR: An venus hystericarum
     unica medela? Reims 1688 (15).

108 BOURDELIN, LUDIVICUS-CLAUDIUS – Prof. FRANC. PICOTÉ DE BELESTRE: An
     amor ingenium mutat? Paris 1717 (14).

109 BOURGAUD, ANT. – Prof. F. MANDAT: An melancholiae et epilepsiae mutuae
     vices? Paris 1650 (14).

110 BOURGAUT, JOHANNES ANT. – Prof. DIONYSIUS GUERIN: An melancholici bre-
     vioris vitae? Paris n. d. (14).

111 BOWER, JOHANNES: De affectione hypochondriaca. Utrecht 1688.

112 BOWITZ, JOHANNES CASPAR – Prof. CHRISTOPH SCHELHAMMER: De catalepsi.
     Jena 1650 (6, 9).

113 BRAAK, SIMON: De catalepsi. Leyden 1693 (8, 9).

114 BRAIER, NICOLAUS – Prof. JACOBUS CORNUTY: An à bile insania? Paris 1626 (14).

115 BRAND, PAULUS – Prof. CLAUS BORRICHIUS: De malo hypochondriaco. Copenhagen 1676 (9, 10, 21).

116 BRAUEL, JOHANNES PHILIPP – Prof. GEORG WOLFFGANG WEDEL: Aeger hypochondriacus illustris medici. Jena 1675 (6).

117 BRAUN, FR. CHR. – Prof. J. MÜLLER: De tarantula. Wittenberg 1676.

118 BRAUN, JEREMIAS JACOB – Prof. JUSTUS VESTI: De suffocatione hysterica. Erfurt 1685 (4, 5, 9, 12).

119 BRAUN, JO. FR. – Prof. EL. CAMERARIUS: Unionis animae cum corpore systemata tria harmoniae praestabilitae, influxus et assistentiae, in unum fusa. Tübingen 1721 (4, 17).

120 BRECHT, CLEMENS JOSEPH – Prof. TOBIAS ANDREAE: De mente et corpore (De conjugio mentis et corporis; De cura mentis per corpus). Frankfurt a. O. 1679 (2).

121 BRECHTFELD, JOHAN. HENR. – Prof. HERMANN CONRINGIUS: De morbo hypochondriaco. Helmstadt 1662 (2, 5, 9, 12).

122 BREMER, E. G. – Prof. R. W. CRAUSIUS: De nymphomania. Jena 1691 (4, 10).

123 BRETSCHNEIDER, JOHANN ADAM: Exhibens aegrum occasione mali hypochondriaci melancholicum. Erfurt 1705 (4, 5).

124 BREYER, L. F. – Prof. RUDOLPH JACOB CAMERARIUS: De potu aquarum ardentium. Tübingen 1698 (17).

125 BREYERUS, GULIELMUS – Prof. ISBRAND DE DIEMERBROECK: De melancholia. Utrecht 1650.

126 BRIENEN, NICOLAUS VAN – Prof. BERNHARD SIEGFRIED ALBINUS: De melancholia. Leyden 1738 (5, 8, 9).

127 BRIOUDE, GABRIEL DE – Prof. GERMANUS PREAUX: An vini quam potus salubrior? Paris 1641 (14).

128 BRUNE, FRIDERICUS WILHELMUS – Prof. JOANN HENR. SCHULZE: Sistens Casus aliquot notabilis aegrotorum mente alienatorum aut perversorum. Halle 1737 (7, 19).

129 BRUNO, BALTHASAR – Prof. GEORG HAMBERGER: De phrenitide. Tübingen 1588.

130 BRUNNER, BALTH.: De phrenitide. Basel 1576 (1, 7, 13).

131 BRUNSCHWITZ, JOHANNES GEORGIUS – Prof. GEORG ERNESTUS STAHL: De impostura opii. Halle 1708 (2).

132 BRUXIUS, CASP.: De melancholia hypochondriaca. Basel 1604 (1, 4).

133 BRUYN VAN BERENDRECHT, DE: De phrenitide. Leyden 1657 (8).

134 BUCHER, URBANUS GOTHOFREDUS – Prof. ADAM BRENDEL: De catalepsi. Wittenberg 1700 (4, 5, 12).

135 BUCHOLTZ, THEODOR GOTTLIEB – Prof. ANDREA ELIAS BÜCHNER: Sistens furorem uterinum. Halle 1747 (2, 5, 9).

136 BUDAEUS, GOTTLIEB – Prof. CHRISTIAN VATER: De natura et cura memoriae. Wittenberg 1686 (4, 5, 9).

137 BÜCHING, GODOFREDUS – Prof. FRIDERICUS HOFFMANN: De potentia diaboli in corpora. Halle 1703 (2, 4, 10, 13).

138 BÜCHNER, ANDREAS ELIAS: De atrocissimo sequioris sexus flagello s. passione hysterica. Erfurt 1721 (5, 9).

139 BÜHREN, DAVID FRIEDRICH: Sistens aegram suffocatione uterino laborantem. Erfurt 1698 (4, 5, 9).

140 BUELIUS, LUDWIG GOTHOFREDUS – Prof. JOHANN JACOB WALDSCHMID: De mania vulgo. Die Tobsucht oder wahnwitzigkeit. Marburg 1680 (2, 4–6, 13).

141 BUENGER, ANDREAS CAROLUS – Prof. ANDREAS ELIAS BÜCHNER: De consensu morborum capitis et ventriculi. Halle 1748 (5).

142 BUGGES: De magia daemoniaca seu illicita, et naturali seu licita. Wittenberg 1667.

143 BULFINGER, BERNARD: De harmonia animi et corporis humani praestabilita. Tübingen 1721.

144 BULISIUS, JOANNES EPHRAIM – Prof. CHRISTIAN GOTTFRIED STENTZEL: De insana sanitate. Wittenberg 1740 (7, 19).

145 BUNTSCH AMBROSIUS GUILIELMUS DE – Prof. JOH. AND. FISCHER: De temperamentorum morumque convenientia et usu medico. Erfurt 1725.

146 BURCHARDUS, CHRISTOPH MARTIN – Prof. GÜNTHER CHRISTOPH. SCHELHAMMER: De morbis magicis. Kiel 1704 (9, 17).

147 (BURCHARDUS, CHRISTIAN MARTIN): De affectione hysterica. Rostock 1718 (17).

148 BURCKHARDT, JOH. RUD.: De melancholia. Basel 1660 (17, 13).

149 BURCKHARDT, CHRISTOPH: De hypochondriaca passione. Basel 1630 (1, 13).

150 BUREN, DANIEL VAN: De affectione hypochondriaca. Leyden 1711 (2, 8, 9, 23).

151 BURGAND, J. ANT. – Prof. FR. MANET: Est melancholiae et epilepsiae mutuae vires. Paris 1650 (14).

152 BURGHARD, J. CHRISTIAN – Prof. G. E. HAMBERGER: De opio. Jena 1749.

153 BURGHART, CHRISTOPH. GEHR. – Prof. CHRISTIAN VATER: De malo sic dicto hypochondriaco. Wittenberg 1703.

154 BUSCH, HENRICUS VAN DEN: De delirio. Leyden 1668 (2, 8, 9).

155 BUSSIUS, AUG.: De imaginationis viribus medicis. Leyden 1698.

156 BUSSIUS, AUG. FRID.: De passione hysterica. Leyden 1692 (23).

157 BUVARDUS, CAROLUS – Prof. JAC LAETUS: An mulieri quam viro Venus Aptior? Paris 1604 (14).

158 BYSCHER, IOANNES GODOFREDUS – Prof. LAURENTIUS HEISTER: De perturbatione animi atque corporis. Helmstadt 1738 (7).

159 CAPAULIS, HERCULES à: De melancholia hypochondriaca. Leyden 1665 (2, 8, 9).

160 CARSTENS, JOHANN GOTTFRIED – Prof. GEORG ERNST STAHL: De empeiria rationali medica. Halle 1704 (17).

161 (CARTHEUSER, JOHANN FRIEDRICH): De noxa et utilitate ebrietatis. Frankfurt a. O. 1740.

162 CASAMAJOR, ANTONIUS – Prof. GABRIELE-ANTONIO JACQUES: An ex negato veneris usu morbi? Paris 1722.

162a CASELIUS, FRID. GOTTH. – Prof. JOHANN ANDREAS FISCHER: De religiosorum sanitate tuendam et restituenda. Erfurt 1721 (4).

163 CASTELLI, GEORG IGNATIUS – Prof. HERMANN PAUL JUCH: De malo hypochondriaco. Erfurt 1745 (6, 7).

164 CELLARIUS, H. – Prof. WERNER ROLFINCK: De affectu hypochondriaco. Jena
1671 (4, 13a).

165 CHASTELAIN, PETRUS: Quaestiones medico-chymico-practicae duodecim. Montpellier 1697 (2).

166 CHAUVEL, RENATUS – Prof. FRANCISCUS PIJART: An ex animi pathematis sani-
tas? Paris 1673 (14).

167 CHAUVEL, RENATUS – Prof. GABRIELE DACQUET: An venus hystericarum medela? Paris 1674 (14).

168 CHEMITIUS – Prof. WERNER ROLFINCK: De melancholia et mania. Jena 1635
(4, 13a).

169 CHOMBART, J.: De mania. Utrecht 1649 (4).

170 CHOMEL, JOANNES-BAPTISTA – Prof. GERMANUS PREAUX: Quaestio Medica.
An omnes Animi Passiones, exceptâ moderatâ Latitiâ, Sanitati noceant? Paris
1731 (14).

171 CHUNO, PHILIPP HENRICUS – Prof. JOHANN JACOB WALDSCHMIDT: Monita
Medica circa opii et opiatorum usum vulgo Schlaff-Tränck. Marburg 1679
(13).

172 CLACIUS, GEORG – Prof. G. E. STAHL: De therapia passionis hypochondriacae.
Halle 1713 (6, 9, 12, 20).

173 CLAUDERUS, GABRIEL – Prof. JOHANN MICHAELIS: De philtris. Leipzig 1661 (2).

174 CLAVILLART, LAURENTIUS: De ira noxa atque ejus utilitate exercitatio phisico-
medica. Montpellier 1744 (2, 11).

175 CLEMENS, JOHANNES FRIDERICUS – Prof. JOHANN FRIEDRICH DEPRÉ: De melancholia hysterica. Erfurt 1727 (2, 4, 12).

176 CLINTH, JOACHIMUS – Prof. JOHANNES PASCHIUS: De fascino per visum et vocem. Wittenberg 1684 (6, 9, 17).

177 CLOOTHACK, MARCUS: De catalepsi. Leyden 1687 (8).

178 CLOSE, SIGISMUND – Prof. GEORG WOLFFGANG WEDEL: De spiritu vini. Jena
1697.

179 COLERUS, JACOB: De scorbuto et hypochondriaca adfectione flatulenta. Basel
1608 (1).

180 COLLOT, ARMANDUS JOSEPHUS – Prof. GERMANUS PREAUX: An morborum den-
tur curationes magneticae? Paris 1696 (14).

181 COMBACHIUS, LUDOVICO – Prof. HENRICUS PETRAEUS: De phrenitide. Marburg
1615 (9).

182 CONRADIUS, J.: De autochiria. Altdorf 1627 (4).

183 (CONRINGIUS, HERMANN): De incantatione circa morbo efficacia. Helmstadt
1659.

184 CONSTANT, PETRUS – Prof. PETRUS SEGUYN: An hystericis quibuscumque
venae sectio? Paris 1636 (14).

185 COOGHEN, ADRIAN VAN DER – Prof. JOAN. WALAEUS: De melancholia hypochondriaca. Leyden 1642.

186 CORBEIUS, HERMANN – Prof. HERMANN CONRINGIUS: De phrenitide. Helmstadt
1645 (2).

187 CORCHWITZ, GEORG DANIEL – Prof. JOH. ERNESTUS STAHL: Reguisita medico at praxin felicem summe necessaria. Halle 1718 (4).

189 CORFINIUS, SIMON: De catalepsi. Utrecht 1669.

190 CORVINUS, JOHANNES FRIDERICUS – Prof. MICHAEL ALBERTI: De potestate diaboli in corpus humanum. Halle 1725 (5, 9).

191 COTTWIZ, JOH. – Prof. DUNCAN LIDDEL: De causis symptomatum principis facultatis. Helmstadt 1598 (13a).

192 (CRAUSIUS, RUDOLF WILHELM): De philtris. Jena 1704.

193 CRELL, A. G. L. – Prof. HERMANN PAUL JUCH: De melancholia hypochondriaca. Erfurt 1737.

194 CRELLIUS, JOHANNES FRIDERICUS – Prof. POLYCARP GOTTLIEB SCHACHER: De melancholia hysterica. Leipzig 1732 (2, 4, 6, 9).

195 CROESER, JACOB: De uteri suffocatione. Leyden 1650.

196 CRÜGNER, L. M. – Prof. J. A. FISCHER: Materia perlata, das ist, edle und bewehrte Artzney wider malum hypochondricum, Miltzkrankheit oder windige Melancholey genannt. Erfurt 1712.

197 CRUSCHIUS, MELCHIOR – Prof. JAKOB HORST: De memoria bona conservanda. Wittenberg 1609 (9, 13a).

198 CRUSIUS, CHRISTIAN ALEXANDER: De superstitione. Leipzig 1741.

199 CRUSIUS, WOLFGANG: De melancholia hypochondriaca. Erfurt 1645 (4).

200 CUMMIUS, JOHANNES CHILIANUS – Prof. RUDOLF WILHELM CRAUSIUS: De delirio in genere. Jena 1686 (4, 6).

201 CUNO, JOHANNES – Prof. DANIEL MOEGLING: De phrenitide. Halle 1584 (4).

202 CURTIUS, ARNOLD – Prof. JOHANN JACOB WALDSCHMIDT: De ebrietate, et insolentibus aliquot ejus effectibus. Giessen 1677 (13).

203 CZAPLINIUS, SAM: De sanitate hominis, cum appendicula de phrenitide. Basel 1619 (1).

204 DANNENBERGER, JOHANNES – Prof. ELIAS CAMERARIUS: Temerarii circa magica judicii exemplum. Tübingen 1729 (5, 16).

205 DAUM, CASPAR CONRAD: De amore insano. Leyden 1704 (8).

206 DEDIER, ANT.: An catalepsia hydragoga? Montpellier 1713 (11).

207 DELARBRE, JOANNES-CLAUDIUS – Prof. PETRUS DE LAURENCEAU: An ab oculis fascinatio? Paris 1678 (9, 14).

208 DELESTRE, IGANTIUS-LAURENTIUS – Prof. PETRO RIDEUX: An passioni hysterica martialia? Montpellier 1711 (2, 11).

209 DELORME, CAROLUS: An amantes iisdem remediis curentur quibus amentes? Montpellier 1608 (11).

210 (DEUSING, ANTONIUS): De delirio simplici et phrenitide. Groningen 1658 (23).

211 DEVILLE, ISAACUS: An catalepsi hydragoga? Montpellier 1713 (11).

212 DEXBACH, AEGIDIUS: De affectione hypochondriaca. Basel 1665 (1, 13).

213 DIDERICH, A. CHR.: De passione miserere mei. Leyden 1703 (8, 19).

214 DIDIER, JACOBUS: An melancholia tum ratione coloris atri an ratione frigiditatis timorem et tristitiam inducat? Montpellier 1629 (11).

215 DIDYMUS, EMAN. – Prof. THEOD. ZWINGER: De phrenitide. Basel 1583 (1, 8).

216 DIETZIUS, PHILIP HENRICUS – Prof. MICHAEL HEILAND: De phanthasia. Giessen 1664 (2).

217 DINTER, HERM. VAN: De phrenitide vera. Leyden 1737 (8).

218 DOLAEUS, J. – Prof. GEORG FRANCUS: De suffocatione hypochondriaca seu
     hysterica. Heidelberg 1673 (4).

219 DORIGNY, ANNA CLAUDIUS – Prof. NATALI. MARIA. DE GEVIGLAND: An a poti-
     bus spirituosis praematura senectus? Paris 1749 (14).

220 DOSE, CONRADUS: De phrenitide. Leyden 1671 (8).

221 DOWNES, JOHANNES: De affectione hypochondriaca. Leyden 1660 (8, 9).

222 DRECHSLER, JOHANN. GABR. – Prof. ADAM RECHENBERG: De spectris. Leipzig
     1668.

223 DU CHEMIN, PETRUS – Prof. JOANNE LE PESCHEUR: An insanienti Virgini Ve-
     nus? Paris 1576 (14).

224 DU MESNIL, JOANNES – Prof. PETRUS LEGIER: An melancholici mollius pur-
     gandi? Paris 1681 (9, 14).

225 DU MOND, JANUS: De hypochondriacorum morbosis affectibus. Utrecht 1705
     (2, 18).

226 DUPONT, MICHAEL – Prof. NICOLAUS CRESPON: An curandis morbis amuleta?
     Paris 1643 (14).

228 DU PRÉ, CAROLUS – Prof. CASPARE BRAYER: An pueris macies à fascino?
     Paris 1630 (14).

229 DUVERNOY, JEAN GEORGE: Theoria vaporum uterinorum, seu pathologia mor-
     bi hysterici. Basel 1710 (1, 13).

230 DYCK, CORNELIUS VAN: De suffocatione hypochondriaca. Leyden 1665 (2, 8).

231 DYLMAN, J.: De phrenitide. Leyden 1654 (8).

232 ECHLITIUS, MAURITIUS CHRISTIANUS – Prof. JOHANN PHILIPP EYSEL: Exhibens
     paraphrenitidem. Erfurt 1710 (5).

233 ECKARD, HIER. – Prof. GEORG WOLFFGANG WEDEL: De terrore. Jena 1697 (5,
     13, 17).

234 (EHINGER, C. C.): De melancholia. Wittenberg 1702. De delirio febr. phreni-
     tis dicto. Wittenberg 1721.

235 (EHINGER, C. C.): De memoriae et capitis laesione a colica spasmodica malo
     curata. Wittenberg 1722.

236 EHRLICH, HIERONYMUS CHRISTIANUS – Prof. FRIDR. HOFFMANN: De affectione
     hypochondriaca. Jena 1652 (12).

237 ELLAIN, NICOLAUS – Prof. PETRUS TOUZET: An hystericis Venus? Paris 1570
     (14).

238 ELNBERGER, ADAMUS HENRICUS: De passione hysterica dem Aufsteigen der
     Mutter. Duisburg 1695 (2).

239 ELWERTH, JOH. PHILIPP – Prof. FRIDER. CHRISTIAN WINCLER: Casus curati
     phrenetici. Heidelberg 1678 (2, 4, 19).

240 EMERY, ANTONIUS-JOSEPHUS – Prof. ANTONIUS MAGNOL: Pro primâ appolinari
     laureâ consequendâ sub hac verborum serie. An mania a sanguinis rarescen-
     tia? Montpellier 1713 (2, 11).

241 EMMEREZ, GUYDO ERASMUS – Prof. AEGIDUS LE BEL: An ab animi pathematis
     sanitas deterior? Paris 1681 (14).

242 ENGELBRECHT, PETRUS CHRISTIANUS – Prof. CHRISTOPH SCHULTZ: De chiro-
     mantiae vanitate. Königsberg 1691 (2).

243 ENGELHAUPT, JOHANNES SIGISMUND – Prof. WERNER ROLFINCK: De dolore capitis, vertigine et phrenitide. Jena 1635 (13a, 17).

244 ENGUEHARD, ANDREAS – Prof. HENRY MAHIEU: An melancholius animi motus vehementiones? Paris 1676 (9, 14).

245 ERDMANN, FRIDERICUS ANDREAS: De passione hysterica strangulatoria. Jena 1710.

246 ERING, A. F. – Prof. J. J. GEELHAUSEN: De viribus imaginationis. Prague 1724.

247 ERMELIUS, JOH. FRID. – Prof. JO. ANDR. FISCHER: De osculo vim philtri ex serente. Erfurt 1719 (2).

248 ESCHENBACH, JOHANNES – Prof. J. RICKEMANN: De satyriasi et priapismo. Jena 1670 (4).

249 ESMARCH, HENRICUS CHRISTIANUS – Prof. JOHANN NICOLAUS PECHLIN: De phrenitide. Kiel 1681 617).

250 ESTH, CASP. – PROF. NIC. TAURELLUS: De melancholia. Basel 1577 (1).

251 FABER, ANTONIUS THEODOR – Prof. JO. MICH. VERDRIES: Aequilibrium mentis et corporis. Giessen 1712 (7).

252 FABIGER, JOHANNES – Prof. SAMUEL POMARIUS: De noctambulis. Dissertatio I. Wittenberg 1649 (6, 9, 12).

253 FABRI – Prof. ANDREAS PLANER: De morbo saturino seu melancholia. Tübingen 1593 (17).

254 FABRICIUS, HIERON.: De mania. Basel 1595 (1, 4).

255 FABRICIUS, JOH. GEORG: De phrenitide. Basel 1620 (1, 13).

256 FABRICIUS, JOHANN PHILIPP – Prof. JOHANN JACOB WALDSCHMIDT: Astrologus Medicus. Marburg n.d. (13).

257 FABRICIUS, WOLFGAANG AMBROSE – Prof. J. G. SALZMANN: De lycanthropia. Strasbourg 1649.

258 FALCKNER, JACOBUS – Prof. DAN. SENNERT: De suffocatione uterina. Wittenberg 1660 (9).

259 FARUS, CHRISTOPH: De melancholia. Leyden 1653 (8).

260 FASCH, AUGUST HENRICUS: De suffocatione uterina. Jena 1680 (6, 17).

261 FAUSTUS, J. WILHELMUS – Prof. WERNER ROLFINCK: Ordo et methodus cognoscendi praecavendi et curandi maniam. Jena 1666 (4, 6, 13a, 17).

262 FELDNER, CASPAR: De suffocatione uteri. Altdorf 1661 (2, 4).

263 FERBER, JOHANN JACOB – Prof. WOLFGANG TRAPPANEGER: Exercitatio academica medicinae mentis. Joachim Langil opposita Strasbourg 1709.

264 FERCKEL, FRANC. LUDOVIC: De deliriis. Strasbourg 1746.

265 FERNANDEZ, PETR.: De praecipuis cerebri affectibus. Leyden 1702 (8, 19).

266 FERRAND, JOANNES BAPTTISTA – Prof. JACOBUS COUSINOT: An ut corporis, sic animi morbis medicina medetur? Paris 1626 (9, 14).

267 FICK, DIETERICUS CHRISTOPH – Prof. HIERONYMUS PHILIPPUS LUDOLFF: De malo hypochondriaco et hysterico incolis Saxoniae inferioris proprio. Erfurt 1725 (2, 7).

268 FICK, JOHANNES JUSTUS – Prof. JOHANN JACOB FICK: De irae efficacia et remediis. Jena 1718 (2, 9).

269 FINCKENAU, JAC. – Prof. CAR. JAC. ROESER: De phanthasiae efficacia in corpus humanum. Königsberg 1705.

270 FINXIUS, DAVID – Prof. JOHANN SIGFRID: De melancholia. Helmstadt 1607 (2).

271 FISCHER, DANIEL – Prof. CHRISTIAN VATER: De deliriis. Wittenberg 1716 (6).

272 FISCHER, H.: De suffocatione uterina. Leyden 1675.

273 FISCHER, JOHANN ANDREAS – Prof. JUSTUS VESTI: De magnetismo macro- et microcosmi. Erfurt 1687 (4, 5).

274 FISCHERUS, J. B. – Prof. JACOB VALLAN: De mania. Utrecht 1709 (5, 12, 18).

275 FISCHER, JOHANN CHRISTOPHER – Prof. L. F. JACOB: De malo hypochondriaco. Erfurt 1713.

276 FISCHER, JO. CONRAD – Prof. FRIDERICH HOFFMANN: Explanatio adfectus maniaci levioris rarissimo sensuum quorundam augmento stipati. Halle 1734 (6, 12, 13, 19).

277 FLACHT, FRIEDR.: De melancholia et idiopathica et sympathica. Basel 1620 (1, 3, 13).

278 FLEISCHER, JOHANNES – Prof. ANSAGARIUS ANCHERSON: De medicatione per musicam. Diss. secundo. Copenhagen 1721 (15, 21).

279 FLOND, AMAND – Prof. RAOUL LELARGE (author): An melancholici prudentiores? Reims 1684 (15).

280 FOCKY, JU. IGNAT: De mania. Wien 1690 (1).

281 FOUCAULT, TOUSS. – Prof. CYPR. HYBAULT: An irasci senibus salubre? Paris 1646 (14).

282 FOUQUÉ, FRANCISCUS – Prof. PETRUS SAVARE: An melancholicorum in medendo praestantior angchinoia. Paris 1625 (14).

283 (FRANCUS DE FRANCKENAU, GEORG): De suffocatione hypochondriaca. Heidelberg 1673.

284 FREHER, C. JOACH.: De melancholia hypochondriaca. Basel 1677 (1, 4, 13).

285 FRENS A LOSTADT, TOBIAS DE – Prof. ISENBRAND DE DIEMERBROECK: De melancholia hypochondriaca. Utrecht 1650.

286 FRIEDERICH, GÜNTHER – Prof. CHRISTIAN LANGE: De malo litteratis familiari sive hypochondriaco. Leipzig 1658.

287 FRIEDERICUS, JOHANN WOLFFGANG: Sistens melancholiam vulgo Die Schwermüthigkeit. Erfurt 1728 (2, 7, 12).

288 FRIEDEBORN, HENRICUS – Prof. GEORG LOTHUS: De morborum literatorum affectus hypochondriacus. Königsberg 1631 (1, 2).

289 FUCHS, DAVID CASPAR – Prof. JOHANN ANDREAS FISCHER: De furore uterino. Erfurt 1724 (2, 6, 7, 12).

290 FUCHS, JOHANNES CONRADUS – Prof. JOH. ARNOLD FRIDERICI: De melancholia. Jena 1671 (4, 5, 10, 17, 19).

291 FÜRST – Prof. ECCARDUS LEICHNER: De mania. Erfurt 1674.

292 FURICHIUS, JOH. NIC.: De phrenitide. Strasbourg 1628.

293 GAEL, IOHANNES: De suffocatione uterina. Leyden 1655 (8, 10).

294 GAETKE, JOA. PETR. – Prof. GE. E. STAHL: De vena portae, porta malorum hypochondriaco-splenico-suffocativo-hysterico-colico-haemorrhoidariorum. Halle 1705 (published 1698).

295 GAILLARD, JOANNES – Prof. JOANNE POISSON: An Amor ingenium mutat? Paris 1695 (14, 9).

296 GALIEN, CLAUDIUS – Prof. THOMAS LE FRICQUE: Utrum comitialibus vita coelebs? Reims 1688 (15).

297 GALON, JAC. FRANC.: De phrenitide. Leyden 1712 (4).

298 GAMARE, JACOBUS – Prof. JOANNE MAURIN: An heroes melancholici? Paris 1646 (14).

299 GAMARE, PETRUS – Prof. AEGIDIUS LE BEL: An animi morbis medicina? Paris 1669.

300 GAMBS, JOH. FRIEDR.: De phrenitide. Basel 1694 (1, 13).

301 GARNIER, GUIDO-ANDREAS – Prof. ELIA COL DE VILARS: An melancholia musica? Paris 1737 (4, 9, 14).

302 GASTALDI, J. BAPT.: De somnambulis. Avignon 1713.

303 GAVIUS, CHRISTIANUS PIUS – Prof. JUSTO VESTI: De passione hysterica. Erfurt 1685 (5).

304 GEBHARD, JOBUS CHRISTIAN – Prof. MICHAEL ERNST ETTMÜLLER: De ira. Leipzig 1705 (2, 6, 12).

305 GEHREN, GEORG ERHARD VON – Prof. GEORG DETHARDING: Scrutinium medicum de morbis a spectrorum apparitione oriundis. Von Gespenstern, wie weit solche durch ihre Erscheinung Kranckheiten verursachen. Rostock 1729 (2, 6, 10, 17, 19).

306 GEILFUS, JOHANN GOTTFR. – Prof. JOHANN DANIEL HORST: De melancholia. Marburg 1643 (22).

307 GEISELBRUNNER, ELIAS: De suffocatione. Basel 1622 (1, 3, 13).

308 GEISENDÖRFFER, BALTH. – Prof. EMAN. STUPANUS: De humanae mentis facultatibus. Basel 1660 (1, 13).

309 GENESTE, ANTONIUS BARTHOLOMAEUS DE LA: De morbo hypochondriaco. Leyden 1673 (2).

310 GENETTE, ANTON CASPAR DE LA: De mania exquisita. Leyden 1723 (8).

311 GENIUS, MICHAEL – Prof. FRANCISCUS DE LE BOË SYLVIUS: De melancholis hypochondriaca. Leyden 1669 (2, 7, 10).

312 GENSELIUS, CHRISTIAN FRID. – Prof. JOHANN ANDREAS FISCHER: Proponens vim fascini in corpus humanum medica arte de victam. Erfurt 1725.

313 GERARDUS, JOANNES: De tristitia. Leyden 1665 (8, 19).

314 GERBER, CHRISTIAN GOTTLOB – Prof. JOHANN PHILIPP EYSEL: De melancholia hypochondriaca. Erfurt 1715 (2, 4, 5, 10).

315 GERDES, JO. – Prof. JER. LOSS: Morborum ab imaginatione ortorum alias idealium idea. Wittenberg 1680 (9, 10).

316 GERHARD, TIDDUS: De suffocatione uterina. Groningen 1703 (5, 23).

317 GERING, P. – Prof. ANDREAS ELIAS BÜCHNER: De causis anxietatis aegrotantium. Halle 1747 (9).

318 GERITS, M. – Prof. MARTIN VON DREMBACH: De phrenitide. Leipzig 1571.

319 GERRESHEIM, ADOLPH FRIED. – Prof. IRENAEUS VEHR: Delirium ex ventriculo. Frankfurt a. O. 1682 (2, 4, 5).

320 GESENIUS, CHRISTIAN: De malo hypochondrico. Utrecht 1704 (18).

321 GESENIUS, GEORGIUS: De suffocatione uterina. Leyden 1654 (8).

322 GIERING, PHILIPP SAMUEL – Prof. LAURENTIUS THEOPHIL. LUTHER: De delirio. Erfurt 1731 (6, 7).

323 GIESWEIN, JOHANNES PHILIPP – Prof. LAURENTIUS STRAUSSIUS: De suffocatione uterina. Giessen 1665 (2).

324 GIGAS, JOH. – Prof. JOH. NIC. STUPANUS: De oblivione seu laesa memoria. Basel 1602 (1).

325 GILGIUS, GEORG WOLFFGANG: De memoriae laesione ex nimio veneris usu oriunda. Altdorf 1691 (4, 17).

326 GILLENIUS, ARNOLD: De phrenitide. Basel 1609 (1, 13, 18).

327 GILPIN, RICH.: De hysterica passione. Leyden 1676.

328 GLADBACH, JO. ADOLPHUS – Prof. JO. PHIL. EYSEL: De ebrietate assidua hydropis causa. Erfurt 1701 (2, 12).

329 GLADEBUSCH, SAM. VALENTIN – Prof. CHRISTOPH HELWIG: De affectione hypochondriaca. Greifswald 1685.

330 GLASBERG, JOD.: De phrenitide. Basel 1591 (1, 13).

331 GLOCK, JOHANNES GEORGIUS – Prof. ELIAS RUDOLPHUS CAMERARIUS: De catalepsi-epileptica. Tübingen 1690 (4, 5).

332 GLOCKENGIESSER, W. TH. – Prof. MICHAEL ALBERTI: Casus menstrui fluxus animalis animique pathematibus perturbati. Halle 1741 (9).

333 GLOSEMEYER, JO. – Prof. A. H. FASCHIUS: De febre amatoria. Jena 1689.

334 GLOXIN, FRIDER. WILHELMUS – Prof. MICHAEL ALBERTI: De autocheiria occulta. Halle 1724 (2, 5, 6, 13).

335 GLUCKIUS, JOHANN ANDREAS – Prof. JOHANN ANDREAS FISCHER: De furore uterino. Erfurt 1720 (2, 4, 7, 9, 19).

336 GLÜCK, FRIDERICUS GOTHOFREDUS – Prof. JOHANN GOTHOFREDUS BERGER: De mania. Leipzig 1685 (4, 5, 9, 10).

337 GLÜTH, JOACHIMUS – Prof. JOHANNES FASCHIUS: De fascino per visum et vocem. Wittenberg 1684 (6).

338 GLYTZ, JOHANN GEORG – Prof. FRIDERICUS HOFFMANN: Morbum convulsivum à viso spectro. Halle 1682 (5, 6).

339 GOCLENIUS, RUDOLPH: Aphorismorum chiromanticorum tractus. Licha 1597 (22).

340 GODARD, GUILLAUME-LAMBERT-DIEUDONNE – Prof. J.-J. BERNARD: De melancholia cephalica. Reims 1745 (15).

341 GODDARD, JACOB: De animi perturbationibus. Leyden 1735.

342 GÖHRS, JOHANNES CHRISTIAN – Prof. MICHAEL ALBERTI: De ebrietate foeminarum. Von Versoffenen Weibes-Personen. Halle 1737 (2, 5).

343 GOLDNER: De nullitate lycanthropiae. Wittenberg 1664.

344 GORDON GEORGIUS – Prof. HERMANN OOSTERDYCK SCHACHT: De spasmo hysterico. Leyden 1734 (2, 8, 12).

345 GORION, STEPHANUS – Prof. NICOLAUS MARCHANT: An a Melancholia mania? Paris 1600 (14).

346 GOTSIUS, Z. N. – Prof. WERNER ROLFINCK: De apoplexia, catalepsi et lethargo. Jena 1630 (13a).

347 GOTTER, JOHANN.-JACOBUS – Prof. GEORG CHRISTOPHORUS PETRI: De suffocatione uterina. Erfurt 1672 (4, 5).

348 GOTTWALDT, CHRISTOPHORUS: De melancholia hypochondriaca. Leyden 1662 (8, 9).

349 GOUEL, FRANCISCUS – Prof. NICOLAOS BAILLY: An ex insomniis temperamenti cognitio? Paris 1685 (9, 14).

350 GOURRAIGNE, HUGO: Quaestio I: An musica morsûs Tarantula unicum sit remedium. Quaestio X: An incubo habituali, elixir proprietatis paracelsi. Montpellier 1732 (2, 11).

351 GOUT, JOANNES-PETRUS: An catalepsi venae sectio? Montpellier 1713 (11).

352 GRABA, JOH. ANDR.: De affectu hypochondriaco cum symptomatibus scorbuti. Giessen 1608 (4, 6).

353 GRAEBNER, GODOFR. LEBRECHT – Prof. MICHAEL ALBERTI: De melancholia vera et simulata. Halle 1743 (2, 4, 5, 12).

354 GRAEF, THEODORUS VAN DE: De catalepsi. Leyden 1716 (8, 9).

355 GRASIUS, C.: Sist. casum autochiriae. Giessen 1712 (15).

356 GRAUEL, JOH. PHIL. – Prof. GEORG WOLFFGANG WEDEL: De aegro hypochondriaco. Jena 1675 (4).

357 GRIESER, C. H. – Prof. JOH. FRID. CARTHEUSER: De superstitione circa curationes morborum magneticas et sympatheticas. Frankfurt a. O. 1744.

358 GRIFFITH, THOMAS: De affectu hypochondriaco. Leyden 1725 (2, 8).

359 GROSSER, BENJAMIN GOTTLIEB – Prof. JOHANN ANDREAS FISCHER: De homine suam et vitae destructore. Erfurt 1727 (6).

360 GROSSMANN, JOH. HAUBOLD –Prof. IRENAEUS VEHR: De mania. Frankfurt a. O. 1701 (2, 4, 5, 6, 19).

361 GRÜBELIUS, JOHANN GEORG – Prof. WERNER ROLFINCK: De strangulatione uteri. Jena 1672 (4, 17, 20).

362 GRÜNDEL, F. W. – Prof. GEORG WOLFFGANG WEDEL: De epilepsia hysterica. Jena 1676 (6).

363 GRUNTINIUS, ANDRZEJ (ANDREAS): Melancholiae, seu affectuum melancholicorum mirabilium, et curatu dificilum. Cracow 1597 (3).

364 GRUNOV, JO. GOD. – Prof. J. JUNKER: De noxa atque utilitate animi pathematum seu adfectum in medicina. Halle 1745.

365 GUALTHERUS JOHANN – Prof. HENRICUS PETRAEUS: De mania. Marburg 1615 (9).

366 GUERING, FRANC. ANTONIUS: De vini. Strasbourg 1740 (2).

367 GUETTARD, JOANNES-STEPHANUS – Prof. PHILIPP CARON: An senibus vinum: aquâ largiori diluendam. Paris 1741 (9, 14).

368 GUGGER, JOH. JAC. – Prof. JOH. NIC. STUPANUS: Olympia iatrica de hysterica affectione. Basel 1607 (1, 4, 13).

369 GULONIUS, HIERONYMUS – Prof. JOANNE HAUTIN: An melancholia imaginatricis affectus? Paris 1610 (14).

370 GUTERMANN, GEORG, FR. – Prof. ALEXANDER CAMERARIUS: De animi efficacia pathematum in negotio sanitatis et morborum. Tübingen 1725 (4).

371 GUTTBIER, JOHANN CHRISTIAN – Prof. LUDOV. FRID. JACOB: Cerevisiae bonitatem. Erfurt 1704 (2).

372 GUYART, PETRUS PAULUS – Prof. LUDOVICUS GALLOIS: Estne corporis exercitatio omnium saluberrina à gaudio? Paris 1678 (9, 14).

373 HAAG, JOHANN WOLFGANG – Prof. JOHANN ADOLF WEDEL: De passione hysterica. Jena 1733 (4, 6, 9, 12).

374 HAENDTSCHKY, MICHAEL – Prof. CHRISTIAN VATER: De melancholia. Wittenberg 1702 (4, 6, 12).

375 HAGEDORN, CHR. – Prof. J. THEODOR SCHENCK: De mania pueororum a fascino. Jena 1667.

376 HAGEN, JOHANNES CONRADUS – Prof. GEORG EMMERICH: De Febre virginum amatoria ex amore. Königsberg 1708 (2, 12).

377 HAGEN, JOHANNES CONRADUS – Prof. JACOB FINCKENAU: De memoria. Königsberg 1709.

378 HAGHEN, CORNELIUS VAN DER: De melancholia hypochondriaca. Leyden 1715 (2, 4, 6, 12).

379 HAHN, JO. FR. – Prof. SAM QUELLMALZ: De maniacis hydropathes. Leipzig 1748 (10).

380 HAHN, LUDWIG AUGUST – Prof. JOHANN HADRIANUS SLEVOGT: Puerperam suffocationis hypochondriaco-hystericae periculo expositam. Jena 1701 (5, 20).

381 HAHN, SIGISMUNDUS: De melancholia hypochondriaca. Leyden 1689 (8).

382 HAKE, CHRISTIANUS FRIDERICUS – Prof. CHR. VATER: De memoriae et capitis laesione gravissima a colica spasmodica male curata. Wittenberg 1722 (2, 4, 19).

383 HALLAYS, FRANCISCUS – Prof. PETRUS MARAIS: An diluentia, in morbis melancholicis, purgationi praeferenda? Paris 1716 (4).

384 HALEWYN, CORNELIUS: De triplici melancholico delirio. Leyden 1624 (5, 9).

385 HAMBERGER, GEORG: De phrenitide. Tübingen 1588 (17, 20).

386 HAMMIUS, GEORG SEBASTIAN: Autocheriae medicae nonnulla specimina. Jena 1708.

387 HANHART, JOH. ULR.: Exhibens mentis aegritudines. Basel 1736.

388 HANNEMANN, JOH. LUDOV.: De usu et abusu inebriantium. Kiel 1679 (6, 8, 9).

389 HANNIEL, STATIUS IOACHIM – Prof. STEPHANI LE MOYNE: De melancholia hypochondriaca. Leyden 1677 (8).

390 HANOLD, JACOB – Prof. NIC. AGERIUS: De facultate intellectiva animae humanae. Strasbourg 1722.

391 HARDT, HERMANN VAN DER – Prof. J. NIDER: De visionibus ac revelationibus. Helmstadt 1692.

392 HARDUINUS DE S. JACQUES, PHILIPPUS – Prof. NICOLAUS REGNIER: An musica in morbis efficax? Paris 1624 (14).

393 HARDUINUS DE S. JACQUES, GABRIEL – Prof. PETRUS COLLIER: An omni melancholiae cardiaca? Paris 1613 (14).

394 HARDUZENUS DE ST. JACQUES, PHILIPPUS – Prof. NICOLAO ELLAIN: Estne Venus Salubris? Paris 1579 (14).

395 HARE, HEINR. VON: De facultatibus animae humanae. Basel 1598 (1).

396 HARMENS, PETRUS: De suffocatione uterina. Greifswald 1687 (5).

397 HARTUNG: De memoria et oblivione. Leipzig 1620.

398 HARTUNG, JO. CPH.: De superstitione. Jena 1685.

399 HARWECK, ADAM: De adfectu hypochondriaco. Königsberg 1696 (5).

400 HASANUS, JO. – Prof. AD. LUCHTENIUS: De melancholia, disp. prima, in qua de melancholia cerebri primaria et ea quae sit per consensum totius, agitur. Helmstadt 1608 (4).

401 HAYMAN, JOHANNIS GUILIELMUS: De praecipuo literatorum morbo affectu hypochondriaco. Leyden 1732 (2).

402 HEBENSTREIT, JOHANN CHRISTIAN: De homicida delirante ejusque criteriis et poena. Leipzig 1723 (6).

403 HEDENUS, NICOLAUS LEONHARDUS – Prof. GEORG WOLFFGANG WEDEL: De epilepsia hysterica. Jena 1676 (4, 5).

404 HÉDOUIN, SIMON – Prof. GERARD LEFILS: An in morborum curatione agyrtarum remidiis debita fides? Reims 1719 (15).

405 HEGGEMAN, FREDERICUS – Prof. JOHANNIS MUNNICKS: De passione hysterica. Utrecht 1694 (18).

406 HEGNER, JOH. HEINR.: De divinatione ex insomniis commentarium philosophico-medico. Basel 1733 (1).

407 HEIDEGGER, PHIL. CONR. – Prof. FRID. CHRIST. WINKLER: De phrenitide. Heidelberg 1681 (4).

408 HEIM, JOHANN CASPAR – Prof. JOHANN ARNOLD FRIDERICI: De hysteromania. Jena 1666 (2, 4, 10, 17).

409 HEINE, NIC.: De phrenitidis theoria et therapia. Basel 1609 (1, 4, 13).

410 HEINRICIUS, AND. – Prof. JO. HAARTMANN: Daemonologia ex principiis rationis eruenda. Abo 1726.

411 HEINTZE, HENRICUS ANTON – Prof. HERMANN CONRING: De incantatibus circa morbos efficacia. Helmstadt 1659 (9).

412 HEINTZE, JOH. CHRISTOPH. – Prof. GEORG DETHARDINGIUS: De erotomania, von der Krankheit, da man verliebt ist. Rostock 1719 (4, 5, 7, 13, 24).

413 HEISTERBERGK, CAROLUS AUGUSTUS – Prof. CAROLUS FRIDER. KALTSCHMIEDIUS: De virgine nymphomania laborante casus. Jena 1748 (4, 6, 12, 13, 17).

415 HELBIGK, CHRISTIANUS – Prof. JOHANN PHILIPP EYSEL: De cerevisia Erfurtensi. Erfurt 1689 (2).

416 HELD, JOHANNES FREDERICUS – Prof. WERNER ROLFINCK: De phrenitide. Jena 1672 (4, 5, 12, 13a).

417 HELE, HENRICUS – Prof. JOHANNIS VAN MUYDEN: De morbis hypochondriacis et hystericis. Utrecht 1719 (2, 5, 8, 18, 23).

418 HELLWIG, JOHANN FRIDERICH – Prof. GEORG BALTHASSAR MEZGER: De passione hysterica. Tübingen 1677 (17).

419 HELWIG, CHRISTOPH. – Prof. PETRI VON HARTENFELS, GEORG CHRISTOPH.: Virginem chlorosi qua volgu dicitur. Die Jungfernkranckheit, Liebes-Farbe, Liebes-Fieber. Erfurt 1693.

420 HEMSKERK, A.: De animae pathematum efficacia in corpus humanum. Leyden 1734.

421 HENCKEL, JOHANN PHILIPP – Prof. JOANNES FRIDERICUS DE PRÉ: De usu et abusu spiritus vini. Erfurt 1720 (7).

422 HENISCH, PAUL – Prof. ISRAEL SPACHIUS: De memoria. Strasbourg 1600 (4).

423 HERFELT, HENRICUS GERRITSEN: De affectione hypochondriaca. Duisburg 1678 (2).

424 HERMANNUS, BENEDICTUS – Prof. GEORGIUS FRANCUS A FRANCKENAU: De musica. Heidelberg 1672.

425 HERNAEUS, JOANNES – Prof. MICHAEL MARAESIUS: An venus morbos gignat, et pellat? Paris 1546 (14).

426 HERON, CORNELIUS: De servanda sanitate literatorum. Leyden 1740 (1, 8).

427 HERON, FRANC.: Est philtris propinatur amor? Montpellier 1652 (11).

428 HERTZBERG, ANT.: De melancholia hypochondriaca. Rostock 1632 (24).

429 HERVEE, JOAN – Prof. MICHAEL MARES: An Venus morbos gignat et expellat? Paris 1546.

430 HERZOG, NIC. – Prof. CONRAD JOHRENIUS: De affectu hypochondriaco. Rinteln 1706.

431 HESSELBARTH, JOHANN CAROLUS GOTTLIEB – Prof. ELIAS ANDREAS BUECHNER: Sistens pathologiam et therapiam passionis hystericae. Erfurt 1739 (5).

432 HEYDENREICH, JUSTUS RUDOLPH – Prof. GEORG WOLFFGANG WEDEL: Proponens juvenem melancholia laborantem (Jüngling mit Melancholie). Jena 1675 (9, 5, 13, 20).

433 HEYL, HEINR.: De melancholia. Basel 1608 (1, 13).

434 HEYLER, Jo. G. – Prof. Jo. ZACCH. PLATNER: On the disease of the ecstatic and diabolically possessed. Leipzig 1732.

435 HEYMAN, JOHANN WILHELM: De praecipuo literatorum morbo affectu hypochondriaco. Leyden 1732 (2, 8).

436 HEYSE, GOTTFRIEDE ERNESTUS: An melancholia balneum? An catalepsi emeticum? Montpellier 1682 (11).

437 HEZEL, DAVID FRANCISCUS – Prof. JOH. JACOB JANTKE: De paralysi et phrenitide. Altdorf 1730 (7, 17).

438 HILDERS, HENRICUS: De generatione spiritus animalis eiusque operationibus et nonnullis capitis affectibus. Leyden 1655.

439 HILSCHER, SIMON PAUL: De philtris. Jena 1704.

440 HIMME, JOH. ERNST – Prof. JOHANN ANDREAS: De strangulatione uteri. Erfurt 1727 (2, 4, 7).

441 HOCHSTETTER, C. L. – Prof. MICHAEL ALBERTI: De remediis morborum superstitiosis. Halle 1737.

442 HOEPPE, JOHANN MARTIN – Prof. MICHAEL ALBERTI: De irae energia ad morbos producendum. Halle 1720 (5).

443 HOERNICAEUS, LUDOVIC: De melancholia natura, differentiis et curatione. Strasbourg 1625 (4, 6).

444 HOFER, JOH. – Prof. JOH. JAC. HARDER: De nostalgia oder Heimwehe. Basel 1688 (1, 10, 17).

445 HOFER, JOHANN: De religiosorum morbis. Basel 1716 (1, 13).

446 HOFMANN, PAULUS – Prof. JOHANN GOTHOFRIED BERGER: De morbis senum. Wittenberg 1693 (17).

447 HOFFMANNUS, CHRISTOPHORUS – Prof. JOHANN ZWINGER: De irae natura, effectibus et remediis. Basel 1699 (1, 4, 13).

448 HOFFMANN, FRIDERICUS – Prof. AUGUSTINUS HENRICUS FASCH: De autoxeipia (Autocheiria). Jena 1681 (4, 6, 9, 10).

449 HOFFMANN, FR., JR. – Prof. FR. HOFFMANN: De morbis hystericis vera indole, sede, origine et cura. Halle 1733 (2, 4, 19).

450 HOFSTETER, JOHANNES CHRISTOPHORUS – Prof. FRIDERICUS HOFFMANN: De animae et corporis commercio. Halle 1695 (2, 4, 6, 7, 9).

451 HOFSTETTER, JOHANNES CHRISTOPHORUS – Prof. FRIDERICUS HOFFMANN: De somnambulatione. Halle 1695 (4, 5, 13).

452 HOMEYER, PAULUS GOTTLIEB – Prof. DAN. MICHAEL ALBERTI: De cerevisiae potu in nonnullis morbis insalubri et adverso, Warum die Kranken das Bier ungern trincken? Halle 1743 (6, 9).

453 HOMMEL, C. FR. – Prof. GEORG GOTTLOB RICHTER: De divinatione. Halle 1744.

454 HOOBROECK, JOHANNES AB: De melancholia. Leyden 1660 (8, 9).

455 HOORN, JOHANNES TE – Prof. BARTHOLOMAEUS DE MOOR: De morbo hypochondriaco. Harderwijk 1715 (2, 20).

456 HORN, J. C. – Prof. WERNER ROLFINCK: De melancholia. Jena 1729 (13a).

457 HORST, GEORG – Prof. TOBIAS TANDLER: De noctisurgio. Wittenberg 1602 (6, 9, 13a).

458 HORST, GREGOR: De mania. Giessen 1677 (2, 4, 5).

459 HOTZELIUS, JOH. GEORG – Prof. NIC. AGERIUS: De anima rationalis. Strasbourg 1626.

460 HOUCK, FR. – Prof. GEORG WOLFGANG WEDEL: De hyperico (alias fuga daemonum). Jena 1716.

461 HOYER, CHRISTOPHORUS EUGENIUS – Prof. MICHAEL ALBERTI: De curationibus sympatheticis. Halle 1730 (2).

462 HUBAULT, CYPRIANUS – Prof. GUILLELMO BELET: An furor amatorius melancholicus affectus? Paris 1621 (14).

463 HÜBNER, JOAN. CHRIST. – Prof. WERNER ROLFINCK: De mania. Jena 1666 (4, 13a).

464 HÜBNER, JOHANN HENRICUS – Prof. IRENAEUS VEHR: De febre virginum amatoria. Frankfurt a. O. 1688 (2, 4, 5).

465 HÜBNER, JOHANN VALENTINUS: De tarantismo. Strasbourg 1674 (2, 16).

466 HUHN, GEORG – Prof. JACOB TAPPIUS: De mania. Helmstadt 1644 (2).

467 HULDENREICH, J. F. – Prof. SAMUEL KALDENBACH: De incubone. Frankfurt a. O. 1656.

468 HUREAU, GERMANUS – Prof. BERTINUS DIEUXIVOYE: An lingua haesitantes melancholici? Paris 1649 (14).

469 HUTH, JOHANN PHILIPP – Prof. MELCHIOR SEBIZIUS: De affecto hypochondriaco. Strasbourg 1651 (2, 16).

470 HUTTEN, JOH.: De phrenitide. Basel 1619 (1).

471 IKEN, H.: De furore uterino, Leyden 1685 (4).

472 IMBERT, GREGORIUS: An aegrotantes imaginarii, sola divessitate idearum, rejecto omni remediorum apparotu, sanandi sint? Montpellier 1723 (11).

473 ITTIG, JOH. FRIEDR. – Prof. MICHAEL ETTMÜLLER: De temulentia. Leipzig 1678 (2).

474 ITTIG, JOHANN – Prof. JOHANNES SCHULTZ: De anima humana. Leipzig 1690 (2).

475 JABOT, NICOLAUS – Prof. GEARDUS DENIZOT: An mania, melancholia, et phrenetis facilius et fiunt ista et curantur? Paris 1586 (14).

476 JACOBI, BALTH. F. – Prof. G. E. STAHL: De morosis aegris, prudentiam medici fatigantibus et flagitantibus. Halle 1714.

477 JACOBI, LUDOVICUS FRIDERICUS – Prof. J. CHR. FISCHER: De malo hypochondriaco. Erfurt 1713.

478 JAEGER, WILHELMUS FRIDERICUS – Prof. ELIAS CAMERARIUS: Medicae quaedam annotationes ad Thomasianum disputationem de praesumptione furoris atque dementiae. Tübingen 1730 (4, 5, 7, 17).

479 JANICHIUS, PETR.: De avante. Basel 1614 (1).

480 JANSSENS, JOHANNIS FRANCICUS: De affectione hypochondriaca. Leyden 1677 (8, 9).

481 JANUS, JACOBUS – Prof. WOLFGANG SCHALLER: De viribus imaginationis. Wittenberg 1624 (1, 9).

482 JACQUEMIN, LUDOVICUS JULIUS – Prof. MICHAEL ALBERTI: De cura per expectationem. Halle 1718 (5, 6).

483 JARVIS, THOMAS: De affectione hysterica. Edinburgh 1744.

484 JENCKE, FRIEDR.: De uteri suffocatione. Basel 1616 (1).

485 JOACHIMUS, JO. – Prof. TOBIAS TANDLERUS: De melancholia ejusque speciebus. Wittenberg 1613 (10, 13a).

486 JÖCHER, C. G. – Prof. MICHAEL ERNST ETTMÜLLER: Affectus musicae in hominem. Leipzig 1714.

487 (JOHRENIUS, J. CONR.): De dolore capitis, phrenitide, melancholia. Rinteln 1674.

488 JONCQUET, DIONYSIUS – Prof. NIC. RICHARD: An Aurora Veneris amica? Paris 1637 (14).

489 JONGH, JOHANNES DE: De uteri suffocatione. Utrecht 1694 (10, 18).

490 JOUVANCY, NICOLAUS DE – Prof. RAYMOND FINOT: An fructus vino temperati salubriores? Paris 1673.

491 JOYEUSE, LUDOVICUS: Exponere theoriam morborum internorum capitis, thoracis et abdominis, absque suppositione spirituum animalium. Montpellier 1720 (11).

492 (JUCH, H. L.): Sistens casum de singulari memoriae imbecillitate ex febre maligna. Erfurt 1731.

493 (JUCH, H. P.): De cognescenda et curanda phrenitide. Erfurt 1745 (7).

494 JUNCKER, JOH.: De phrenitide. Basel 1618 (1, 4).

495 JUNGERMANN, LUDOVICUS – Prof. GREGOR HORST: De curatione vesani amoris. Giessen 1611 (13a).

496 JUSTUS, LUCAS – Prof. JOH. NIC. STUPANUS: De facultatibus animae. Basel 1596 (1).

497 KÄSEBERG, FRIDERICUS – Prof. GEORG WOLFFGANG WEDEL: De morbis a fascino. Jena 1682 (4, 6).

498 KALDENBACH, MELCHIOR BENJAMIN – Prof. IRENAEUS VEHR: De phanthasia morborum parente et medico. Frankfurt a. O. 1681 (4, 6).

499 KALTSCHMIDT, FRIDERICUS FERDIN. – Prof. GEORG WOLFFGANG WEDEL: De phrenitide. Jena 1710 (4, 5, 12).

500 KAMITZERUS, JACOBUS – Prof. JUSTUS VESTI: Sistens aegrum melancholia amatoria, variis symptomatibus gravioribus maritata. Erfurt 1705 (2, 4, 5, 9, 12).

501 KAU, JACOBUS: De malo aphrodisi. Utrecht 1697.

502 KAUFMANN, HERM.: De uteri suffocatione. Basel 1652 (1).

503 KAULITZ, A. C. – Prof. MICHAEL ALBERTI: De commercio animae s. naturae incorporeae, cum medicis et remediis corporeis. Halle 1720 (2).

504 KAULIZIUS, MICHAEL – Prof. GEORG WOLFFGANG WEDEL: De oblivione. Jena 1690 (5).

505 KESSEL, GODOFRIDUS VAN DER: De phrenitide. Leyden 1684 (8).

506 KEIL, ANDREAS – Prof. CONRAD VICTOR SCHNEIDER: De melancholia. Wittenberg 1666 (12).

507 KEIL, PETER PH. – Prof. AUGUST FRIEDRICH WALTHER: De temperamentis et deliriis. Leipzig 1741 (5).

508 KELLER, STEPHANUS – Prof. CHRISTIANUS GOTTFRIED STENTZEL: De poculis sanitatis poculis morborum et mortis. Wittenberg 1738 (7, 9, 10, 17).

509 KEPPEL, WILHELM: De hysterica passione. Utrecht 1710 (18).

510 KETELL, GUIELIELMUS: De passione hysterica. Utrecht 1724 (18).

511 KHIEN, FERDINANDUS – Prof. CONRAD VICTOR SCHNEIDER: De phrenitide. Wittenberg 1666 (9, 12).

512 KHOLBMANN, CONRAD: De uteri strangulatu. Basel 1591 (1).

513 KHONN, ALPHONSUS: De catalepsi. Strasbourg 1662 (2, 4).

514 KIRCHOVIUS, PAULUS: De mentis et animae consensu et dissensu. Leyden 1725 (8).

515 KISNER, JOHANN – Prof. CHRIST. HUNDSHAGEN: De imaginatione ejusque viribus. Jena 1665 (5, 6).

516 KISNER, JOHANNES: De suffocatione hypochondriaca. Leyden 1670 (2, 4, 6, 8, 9).

517 KLEIN, GODOFRIED – Prof. GEORG WOLFFGANG WEDEL: De melancholia. Jena 1707 (2, 4, 5, 8, 12).

518 KLETSCHKE, DAVID GO. – Prof. MICHAEL ALBERTI: De superstitione medica. Halle 1720.

519 KLOCKHOF, CORN. ALB. – Prof. HIER. DAVID GAUBIUS: De morbis animi. Utrecht 1753 (13).

520 KLUG, GE. PHIL. – Prof. GODOFREDUS MOEBIUS: De phrenitide. Jena 1647.

521 KNIPHOF, JOHANN HIERONYMUS: De physiognoma. Erfurt 1737.

522 KNÖVENAGEL, CHN. – Prof. JACOB FABRICIUS: De uterina vel hysterica suffocatione. Rostock 1628 (24).

523 KNOLL, JOHANNES DANIEL – Prof. CHRISTIAN VATER: De delirio febrili phrenitis dicto. Wittenberg 1721 (4, 5, 9).

524 KOCH, DANIEL – Prof. JOANNES FRIDERICUS DE PRÉ: De hyperemesi casu, gravioribus symptomatibus stipata, cum subsequenti delirio. Erfurt 1722 (5).

525 KOCH, JOH. MARCUS: De melancholia hypochondriaca. Strasbourg 1665 (4, 16).

526 KOEBERER, DAVID – Prof. J. CONRAD BRODTBECK: Catalepsis a Galeno descripta. Tübingen 1660 (5).

527 KOHEN, LEHM. ISAAC – Prof. GEORG GOTTLIEB RICHTER: De morbo hypochondriaco. Göttingen 1739.

528 KOHLER, JOHANN REINHARD – Prof. JOHANN RUDOLPH SALTZMANN: De somnambulis. Strasbourg 1651 (4, 12,16).

529 KOKUYT: De melancholia. Leyden 1685 (1, 3).

530 KORNMESSER, JACOB – Prof. CASPAR MARCH: De affectione hypochondriaca. Rostock 1665 (13, 24).

531 KORNZWEIG, JOHANNES HENRICUS PAULUS: De epilepsia a terrore orta. Giessen 1713 (17).

532 KRAHE, PETRUS: De furore uterino. Duisburg 1705 (2).

533 KRAPFF, JOH. WOLFGANG – Prof. JO. NIC. STUPANUS: Positiones iatrica de phrenitide. Basel 1607 (1, 13).

534 KRAUS JOHANN GOTTLIEB – Prof. MELCHIOR SCHEFFER: De phanthasia ejusque affectibus cum applicatione ad fanaticos. Leipzig 1706.

535 KRÖS, ANTONIUS; HETTENBACH, BALTHASAR et CADEMANN, AUGUSTUS – Prof. TOBIAS TANDLER: De matricis praefocatione. Wittenberg 1614 (6, 13a).

536 KRYT, CORNELIUS DE – Prof. CORNELIUS VAN ECK: De hysterica passione. Utrecht 1696 (18).

537 KUHN, JOHANNES: De phrenitide. Utrecht 1663.

538 KÜHNE, CHRISTOPH. FRIDERIC. – Prof. JOH. ADOLPH WEDEL: De phrenitide. Jena 1736 (2, 4, 5, 12, 19).

539 KUESCH, ERICUS – Prof. JOH. ZACHARIAS PLATNER: Medicos de insanis et furiosis audiendos esse, ostendit. Leipzig 1740 (6, 7, 13).

540 KUNADUS, THEODORUS – Prof. JEREMIAS LOSS: Erotomania seu amoris insani. Wittenberg 1681 (5).

541 KURTZ, CAROLUS JOSEPHUS – Prof. HERMANN PAUL JUCH: De ebrietate ejusque noxis praecavendis et tollendis. Erfurt 1741 (2, 6, 7, 9).

542 LAM, JOHANNES – Prof. JAC. VAN WACHENDORFF EVERARD: De phrenitide. Utrecht 1748 (18).

543 LAMAND, JEAN: De natura amoris et amantium amentium cura. Basel 1614 (1, 13).

544 LAMBERTUS, JOH. FRIDERICUS MARQUARD: De Febri amatoria. Leyden 1706 (1, 13).

545 LAME, CHR. – Prof. C. BARTHOLINUS: De memoria. Copenhagen 1693 (21).

546 LAMMERS, GERH.: De phrenitide. Groningen 1666.

547 LA MOTTE, HENR. JAC. DE: De malo hysterica. Strasbourg 1738 (16).

548 LAMY, ALANUS – Prof. JOANNE BOURGEOIS: An phrenitide hypnotica? Paris 1654 (14).

549 LANGE, SAMUEL – Prof. JO. PHILIPP EYSEL: De fuga daemonum. Erfurt 1714 (4, 5).

550 LANGENSTÄTTER, JOHANNES CONRADUS – Prof. JOHANN CONRAD BRUNNER: De affectione hypochondriaca. Heidelberg 1688.

551 LANGGUTH, GE. AUG.: Communis sensorii historiam. Leipzig 1738 (6).

552 LANNOY, ARNOLDUS DE – Prof. ARNOLDI SYEN: De mania. Leyden 1674 (8, 10).

553 LAURENTIUS: De hystericis affectibus, infantilibusque morbis. Leyden 1595 (6).

554 LATIMER, THOMAS – Prof. BERNHARDUS ALBINUS: De somnambulatione. Frankfurt a. O. 1689 (2, 9).

555 LAUNAY, HERMANN DE – Prof. JOANNE HENAULT: An vinum adultis, aqua pueris? Paris 1623 (9, 14).

556 LAUREA, GEORG: De febris melancholicis. Basel 1596 (1, 13).

557 LAURENTIUS, BONIFACIUS – Prof. GUNTH. CHRISTOPH SCHELHAMMER: De obsessis. Kiel 1704 (17).

558 LEAULTÉ, URBANUS – Prof. PETRUS PERREAU: An praecavendis tum corporis tum animi morbis aquae potus? Paris 1686 (9, 14).

559 LE CLERC, ANTONIUS – Prof. AMBROISE NICOLAUS CHEMINEAU: An robur corporis obstat vi et praestantiae intellectûs? Paris 1695 (9, 14, 20).

560 LEDELIUS, SAMUEL: De phrenitide. Jena 1667.

561 LEEUW, JOHANNES DE: De catalepsi. Leyden 1695 (8, 10).

562 LE GAIGNEUR, STEPHANUS – Prof. PETRUS LE COMTE: An daemonas incorpora subeuntes nonnumquam internus calor imitetur? Paris 1638 (14).

563 LEGIER, PETRUS – Prof. LANCELOT DE FRADE: An non Amans, Amens? Paris 1632 (14).

564 LEHMANN, JOANNES MATTHAEUS – Prof. JO. PHILIP EYSEL: De furore uterino, oder Tobsucht der Weiber. Erfurt 1715 (2, 4, 5, 12).

565 LEHMANN, JOANNES MATTHAEUS – Prof. JO. PHILIP EYSEL: De melancholia hypochondriaca. Erfurt 1715 (4).

566 (LEICHNER, ECCARD): Casus Matronae hypochondriacae. Erfurt. 1685.

567 LEISNER, JO. GOTTL. – Prof. JOHANN CHRISTIAN STOCK: De malo hypochondriaco-hysterico. Jena 1749 (4).

568 LE LONG, CAROLUS – Prof. FLORIMUNDO LANGLOIS: Est-ne unquam salubris ebrietas? Paris 1665 (9, 14).

569 LENGRENE, THOMAS: Potestne ebrietas esse salutaris? Montpellier 1647 (11).

570 LEONARDUS, A. G.: Sistens melancholiam hypochondriacam. 1737 (12).

571 LEOPOLD, JOHANN – Prof. JOHANN SIGLICIUS: De melancholia morbo. Leipzig 1613 (4, 9).

572 LE PIPER, JOHANNES – Prof. ELIAS EVERHARD VORSTIUS: De melancholia. Leyden 1621 (2, 8, 9).

573 LEPY, P. A. – Prof. JO. CORDELLE: An vinum alimentum, medicamentum, venenum? Paris 1714 (14).

574 LESPIÈRE JOSEPH-PONCE DE – Prof. JEAN LAPILE: An congressus Daemonis irritus? Reims 1675 (15).

575 LE LETIER, SIMON: An convulsio hysterica encheres? Paris 1618 (14).

576 LE RAT, FRANCISCUS – Prof. PHILIPP MATHON: An opium hystericae accessioni noxium? Paris 1677 (14).

577 LEVIN, ABRAHAM – Prof. MICHAEL ALBERTI: De vi imaginationis in vitam et sanitatem naturalem. Halle 1740 (2).

578 LIDDEL, DUNCAN – Prof. FRANCISIUS PARCOVIUS: De melancholia. Helmstadt 1596 (9, 13a).

579 LINCKE, JOHANN JOACHIM – Prof. IRENAEUS VEHR: De suffocatione hysterica. Frankfurt a. O. 1678 (2, 4, 5).

580 LINPRUNER, JOSEPH ANTONIUS – Prof. JOHANN ANDREAS SEGNER: De paraphrenitide. Göttingen 1747.

581 LIPSTROP, CHRISTOPHORUS: De morbis passionum animi. Leyden 1719 (8).

582 LISCHWITZ, J. CHR. – Prof. MICHAEL ETTMÜLLER: De vitiis circa somnum et vigilias. Leipzig 1720 (13).

583 LOCHNER, MICH. FRIED.: De nymphomania historiam medicam. Altdorf 1689
     (4, 13, 17).
584 LOESCHER, VAL. ERN.: De visionibus et revelationibus. Disp. contra Peterse-
     nium. Wittenberg 1692.
585 LOGAN, GEORG ADAM – Prof. LUDOVIC FRIDERICUS JACOBI: De anima, causa
     morborum proxima. Erfurt 1691 (12).
586 LOHEN, CHRISTOPHORUS A – Prof. DANIEL BECKHER: De phrenitide.
     Königsberg 1639 (4).
587 LOMBARD, PETRUS – Prof. MARTIN AKAKIA: An melancholius meri potio salu-
     bris? Paris 1666 (9, 14).
588 LONER, GABRIEL – Prof. JOHANNES RICKEMANN: ordo et methodus cognoscen-
     di, praecavendi et curandi ebrietatem et inde ortum crapulam. Jena 1670 (4,
     9).
589 LONGIUS, D. H. – Prof. MART. CHLADENIUS: De visionibus Hildegardis. Wit-
     tenberg 1716.
590 LOTHUS, GEORG: De morbo literatorum, qui vulgo affectus hypochondriacus
     indigitatur. Königsberg 1631 (5).
591 LOTICHIUS, JOH. HENRICUS – Prof. JOH. WILHELM HECHLER: De noctambulis.
     Giessen 1665 (12).
592 LOVELL, GUILIELMUS: De febri delira seu delirio. Leyden 1673 (8).
593 LUCIUS, G. PH.: De curis morborum sympatheticis. 1732 (12).
594 LUDOLFF, PHILIPPUS – Prof. GEORG VOLKMAR HARTMANN: De commercio ani-
     mae cum corpore secundum diversas philosophorum hypotheses. Erfurt 1725.
595 LUPICHIUS, FRIEDR.: De risu. Basel 1738 (1).
596 LUSSON, GUIL. – Prof. V. HIERAUME: An mulieri ab utero quam à capite plures
     morbi? Paris 1574 (14).
597 LUTHERITIUS, P.: De noxa et utilitate ebrietatis. Frankfurt a. O. 1740.
598 LY, THEODORUS: De phrenitide. Utrecht 1701 (18).
599 LYSTHENIUS, J. F.: De suffocatione uterina. Jena 1661.
600 MAEDER, THEOPHILUS – Prof. THOMAS ERASTUS: De morbis totius substantiae.
     Basel 1575 (1, 13).
601 MAERCKY, DAVID – Prof. THEOD. ZWINGER: De morbis a fascino, et fascino
     contra morbos pars prior, sistens examen philol.-philosophicum oeconomiae
     spirituum, eorumque in corpora humana potestatis pars prior. Basel 1723 (1,
     4, 7, 13).
602 MAERCKY, DAVID – Prof. THEOD. ZWINGER: De morbis a fascino et fascino
     contra morbos pars posterior. Basel 1723 (1, 4, 7, 13).
603 MAGNY, GUIL. DE – Prof. JAC. JUL. CARRÉ: An quo salacior mulier, eo foe-
     cundior? Paris 1720 (14).
604 MAGNUS, GO. FR. – Prof. CONST. ZIEGRA: De magia. Wittenberg 1665.
605 MAILLY, NICOLAS DE – Prof. JEAN LAPILE: An morbis a maleficio curatio?
     Reims 1667 (15).
606 MAJAULT, MICH. JOS. – Prof. PET. ANT. LEVY: An aqua vitae aqua mortis?
     Paris 1737 (14).
607 MAJUS, HENRICUS – Prof. ANTON. DEUSINGIUS: De somnambulatione. Gronin-
     gen 1657 (12).

608 MAJUS, JOHANNES: De passione hysterica. Utrecht 1692 (8, 9, 18).

609 MALAT, PIERRE – Prof. PIERRE LE PESCHEUR (author): An in morbis melancholicis purgatis per inferiora? Reims 1689 (15).

610 MALEY, JOHANNES GEORGIUS – Prof. GEORGIUS WOLFFGANG WEDEL: Aegrum memoria debilitate laborantem. Jena 1696.

611 MALLET, EUSTACHE – Prof. CLAUDE NOLIN (author): An melancholia morbo laborantibus musica? Reims 1664 (15).

612 MALLINKROTT, A. – Prof. CAROLUS ANDREAE DUKER: Ebrietatis pathologia. Utrecht 1723 (7, 18).

613 MALOT, PIERRE – Prof. PIERRE LE BESCHEUR (author): An in morbis melancholicis purgatio per inferiora? Reims 1689 (15).

614 MALUS: De passione hysterica. Utrecht 1693 (18).

615 MAN, JOHANNES DE: De catalepsi. Leyden 1671 (2, 4, 8).

616 MANGOLDT, JOHANN GEORG: De catalepsi. Basel 1673 (1, 13).

617 MARDORFF, JOH. JACOB: De maniacis. Giessen 1691 (12, 17).

618 MARESCHAL, ANTONIUS ARTUS – Prof. FRANCISCUS DE LE BOË SYLVIUS: Continens casum epilepticum. Leyden 1669 (2).

619 MARQUARD, LAMBERTUS JOH. FRIDERICUS: De febre amatoria. Leyden 1706 (8).

620 MARTINUS, SIGISM. – Prof. ADAM LUCHTENIUS: De phrenitide. Helmstadt 1607 (4).

621 MARTIUS, JOHANNES NICOLAUS: De magia naturalis, eiusque usu medico ad magicae et magica medicae. Erfurt 1700 (2, 5).

622 MARTIUS, THEODORUS – Prof. JO. PHILIPP EYSEL: Exhibens visionis statum naturalem et praeternaturalem. Erfurt 1696.

623 MAST, PASCHASIUS VANDER: De suffocatione uterina. Leyden 1651 (4).

624 MATHIS, JOHANNES CONRADUS: De mania. Strasbourg 1669.

625 MATTHEI, JOHANN BERNHARD – Prof. GEORG FRANCUS: Demens idea s. de mania. Heidelberg 1680 (4, 20).

626 MAUL, CHRISTIANUS – Prof. PAUL GOTTFRID SPERLING: De salacitatis natura et cura. Wittenberg 1701 (6, 9).

627 MAURIN, RAPHAEL – Prof. PETR. PERREAU: An Melancholicis Venus? Paris 1658 (14).

628 MAURIN, R. – Prof. N. LIENARD: An salicitate vita brevior? Paris 1657 (14)

629 MAYR: De passione hysterica. Leyden 1625 (10).

630 MEIER, FRIEDRICH GOTTLIEB – Prof. GEORG GOTTLOB RICHTER: De malo hysterico. Göttingen 1741 (9, 12, 20).

631 MEIERUS, JOH. JACOBUS: Meditatio de memoria laesa seu oblivione. Basel 1687 (1).

632 MEINEKE, A. CHR. – Prof. FR. HOFFMANN: De vera morbi hypochondriaci sede, indole ac curatione. Halle 1719 (20).

633 MEISNER, HENRIC. – Prof. JOH. RUDOLPH SALTZMANN: De noctambulis. Strasbourg 1663.

634 MELANCHTHON, PHIL.: De melancholia hypochondriaca positiones. Basel 1629 (1, 4).

635 MELM, JOHANNES CONRADUS: De catalepsi. Duisburg 1700 (19).

636 MENDEZ DE ALMANSA, ARON: De melancholia. Leyden 1661 (8).

637 MENTZELIUS, JOHANN CHRISTIAN – Prof. BERNHARD ALBINUS: De aegro melancholia hypochondriaca laborante. Frankfurt a. O. 1684 (9).

638 MERCKEL – Prof. BERNARDUS ALBINUS: De aegro melancholia hypochondriaca laborante. Frankfurt a. O. (4).

639 MERZ, PHILIPP PAUL: De imaginatione. Strasbourg 1719.

640 MESCHMANN, JOHANNES HENR. – Prof. FR. HOFFMANN: De animo sanitatis et morborum fabro. Halle 1699 (4, 5, 12).

641 MESMIL, JOANNES DE – Prof. PETRUS LEGIER: An melancholici mellius purgandi? Paris 1681.

642 MEVIUS, THOMAS TOBIAS – Prof. SIMON FRIEDRICH FRENZEL: Ex chiromantia. Wittenberg 1663 (9).

643 (MICHAELIS, JOHANNIS): De affectu hypochondriaco. Leipzig 1634 (4).

644 (MICHAELIS, J.): De phrenitide. Leipzig 1648.

645 MILLER, IOANNES FRIDERICUS WILHELMUS – Prof. HIER. DAVID GAUB: De morbis abusu potus oriundis. Leyden 1743 (8).

646 MINOT, JACOBUS – Prof. FRANCISCO VEZOU: An vires consociae amant opium a Chinâ Chinâ? Paris 1696 (9, 14).

647 MISLER, JOHANN JACOB – Prof. JOHANN JAKOB WALDSCHMIDT: De stupendo illo affectu, catalepsi. Marburg 1678 (6, 13).

648 MITHOBIUS, FRANZ BURKHARD: De catocho seu catalepsi. Basel 1629 (1).

649 MOCHINGER, GEORG: De affectu hypochondriaco. Leipzig 1628.

650 MOEBIUS, GODOFREDUS – Prof. WERNER ROLFINCK: De affectu hypochondriaco. Jena 1640 (13a).

651 (MOEBIUS, GODOFREDUS): De suffocatione uterina. Jena 1661.

652 MOEBIUS, PAULUS CHRISTOPH. – Prof. JOHANN THEODOR SCHENCK: De catalepsi. Jena 1671 (4, 9, 12).

653 MOEGLING, ULR. – Prof. JO. ADAM OSIANDER: De transmigratione animarum humanarum ex suis corporibus in alia corpora. Tübingen 1749.

654 MÖLLERUS, JO. GEORGIUS – Prof. JO. HADRIAN SLEVOGT: De affectibus animi diatribe physiologica. Jena 1695 (12, 19).

655 MOERINGH, ALBERTUS: De animi pathematis. Leyden 1673 (8).

656 MOHR, NICOLAUS CONRAD – Prof. CONRAD JOHRENIUS: De affectu hypochondriaco. Rinteln 1678 (6, 9, 13, 20).

657 MOLEY, J. G.: De aegro memoriae debilitate laborante. Jena 1696.

658 MOLL, THEODORUS: De suffocatione uterina. Utrecht 1662.

659 MOLLER, CAROLUS OTTO: De divino in medicina. Altdorf 1696 (17).

660 MOLLER, D. G.: De terrore panico. Altdorf 1699 (4).

661 MOLSWYCK, IACOBUS – Prof. JOHANNIS HOORNBEEK: De phrenitide. Leyden 1664 (8, 9).

662 MONTIGNY, JOANNES DE – Prof. GUIDO PATIN: Estne longae ac incundae vitae testa certaque parens sobrietas? Paris 1648 (9, 14).

663 MOOR, BARTHOLOMAEUS DE – Prof. FRANCISCUS DE LE BOË SYLVIUS: De suffocatione hypochondriaca. Leyden 1669 (2, 8).

664 MORIAU, PETRUS – Prof. HOMMETZ: An singulis mensibus repetita semel ebrietas salubris? Paris 1643.

665 MORIS, PETRUS – Prof. JOHANNIS COCCIUS: De suffocatione uterina. Leyden 1676 (8).

666 MORISSE, GUILLELMUS – Prof. PETRUS OUDINET: An jocosi sint melioris habitus? Reims 1673 (15).

667 MOSSDORF, J. FRIDERICUS – Prof. MICHAEL ALBERTI: De valetudinariis Imaginariis. Von Menschen die aus Einbildung krank werden. Halle 1721 (4, 6, 9, 10).

668 MOTTE, H. J. DE LA: De malo hypochondriaco. Strasbourg 1738 (16).

669 MOUSTELON, GABRIEL – Prof. JO. ASTRUC: De phantasia sive imaginatione. Montpellier 1723 (9, 11).

670 MUCHE, CHR. – Prof. WERNER ROLFINCK: De phrenitide. Jena 1652 (or Moche).

671 MÜLLER, ALBINUS – Prof. MELCHIOR SEBIZ: De rigore, horrore, refrigeratione, oxitatione, pandiculatione, palpitatione, tremore et dentium stridore. Strasbourg 1653 (16).

672 MÜLLER, JOH. – Prof. AUG. HEINR. FASCH: De febre amatoria. Jena 1689 (4, 5, 9).

673 MÜLLER, ACHATUS – Prof. IRENAEUS VEHR: De astrobolismo. Frankfurt a. O. 1690 (5).

674 MULLER, J. FR. – Prof. H. CH. ALBERTI: Casus pecul. de morbo motuum habituali ex imaginatione sub ructuum schemate enato. Halle 1732.

675 MÜLLER, JAC. FRID.: De lycanthropia seu de transmutatione in lupos. Leipzig 1673.

676 MÜLLER, JOH. B. – Prof. SIMON PAUL HILSCHER: De melancholia. Jena 1727.

677 MULLERUS, JOH. JACOBUS – Prof. HERM. FRIDER. TEICHMEYER: De melancholia attonita raro litteratorum affectu. Jena 1741 (4, 6, 12).

678 MÜLLER, JOHANN JULIUS – Prof. JAC. TAPPIUS: De catalepsi. Helmstadt 1660 (4).

679 MULLERUS, JOANNES PAULUS – Prof. JACOB TAPPIUS: De phrenitide. Helmstadt 1643.

680 MÜLLER, JOHANN ULRICUS: De mania seu insania. Strasbourg 1654 (4).

681 MÜLLER, SAMUEL – Prof. ECCARDUS LEICHNER: De melancholia hypochondriaca. Erfurt 1689 (5).

682 MÜLLER, MATTHAEUS – Prof. SEBASTIAN BLOSSIUS: De phrenitide. Tübingen 1602.

683 MUYS, WYERUS WILHELMUS: De catalepsi. Utrecht 1701 (5, 19).

684 MYLIUS: De maniae theoria et praxi. Giessen 1672 (17).

685 NAEVIS, CAROL. GOTTLOB – Prof. LUD. HENR. HILCHEN: De phrenitide. Giessen 1742 (2).

686 NAGEL, JOSEPH CHRISTIAN: De celebri spectro quod vulgo die weisse Frau nominant. Wittenberg 1723.

687 NAGY, BOROSNYAI MARTINUS – Prof. FRIDERICUS HOFFMANN: De potentia et impotentia animae humanae in corpus organicum sibi junctum. Halle 1728.

688 NAUHEIMER, JOANNES J.: De sobrietate. Erfurt 1741.

689 NEBEL, DANIEL: Quid de methodo Harveana morbos expectatione curandi sit sentiendum. Marburg 1695.

690 NEERINEX, VINCENTIUS: De melancholia. Leyden 1727 (2, 8).

691 NEIDE, AUGUSTUS: De morbis animi. Halle n. d. (2).

692 NEUCRANZ, MICHAEL: De uteri suffocatione. Strasbourg 1632.

693 NEUFFER, CHR. – Prof. ELIAS CAMERARIUS: De magici morbi historia. Tübingen 1724 (5).

694 NEUFVILLE, ISAAC DE – Prof. GEORG OTTO: Miranda vis imaginationis. Marburg 1691.

695 NEUHAUS, GEORG SEBASTIAN – Prof. CHRISTOPH MARTIN BURCHARDUS: De affectione hysterica. Rostock 1718 (2, 4, 12).

696 NEUHOFF, DANIEL GOTTLIEB – Prof. JOHANN PHILIPP: Proponens satyriasis. Erfurt 1710 (1, 2, 4, 7, 9).

697 NEUMANN, CHRISTIAN GOTTLIEB: De exclusione ovulorum in salacibus, absque ullo praegresso coitu. Leyden 1717 (8).

698 NEUSE, JOHANN GEORG – Prof. GEORG WOLFFGANG WEDEL: De melancholia. Jena 1685 (4, 6, 12, 13, 18, 20).

699 NICOLAUS, DANIEL – Prof. BERNHARDUS ALBINUS: De mania. Frankfurt a. O. 1692 (2, 4, 6, 17).

700 NICOLL, SCOTT JOSEPHUS: De quibusdam capitis nervorumque affectionibus. Edinburgh 1744.

701 NIESIUS (NIESS), BENJAMIN: Defensio medica necessaria de affectione hypochondriaca. Frankfurt a. O. 1674.

702 NIETNER, JOHANN GOTTFRIED – Prof. JOHANN PHILIPP EYSEL: De nymphomania. Erfurt 1694 (6).

703 NIFANIUS, CHR.: De lycanthropias figmento. Giessen 1654.

704 NISSEN, CHRISTIAN – Prof. ANSAGARIUS ANCHERSON: De medicatione per musicam (Diss. tertio). Copenhagen 1722 (21).

705 NOEBLING, JOHANN WILHELM – Prof. JOHANN CHRISTIAN STOCK: De cadaveribus sanguisugis, von den sogenannten Vampyren oder Menschensaugern. Jena 1732 (6).

706 NOËL DE PIVIER, NICHOLAS BENJAMIN – Prof. BERNHARD ALBINUS: De tarantismo. Frankfurt a. O. 1691 (5, 10).

707 NOTTELMANN, BERNARDUS ARNOLDUS: De melancholia. Utrecht 1693 (8, 18).

708 NUCELLA, ISAAC: De mania. Utrecht 1697 (18).

709 OBER, CHRISTOPHORUS – Prof. WILHELM HULDER. WALDSCHMIDT: De imaginatione hominum et brutorum. Kiel 1701 (2, 12, 13).

710 OBRECHT, DAN.: De melancholia hypochondriaca. Strasbourg 1581 (4).

711 OCHLITIUS, SAMUEL – Prof. JOH. THEODOR SCHENCK: De passione hypochondriaca. Jena 1666 (10, 12, 20).

712 OCHOCKI, GABRYAL: De phrenitide. Cracow 1629 (3).

713 O'DONOCHOO, ARTHURUS EDMUNDUS – Prof. THOMAS LE FRICQUE: An medicus sit sensualis physicus? Reims 1676.

714 OERTELIUS, IO. ADAM – Prof. HERM. FRIDERICUS TEICHMEYER: De delirantium furore et dementia. Jena 1733 (2, 4, 12).

715 OHM, WILHELMUS – Prof. FRIDER. CHRISTIAN WINKLER: De melancholia specie qui affectae pro sagis vulgo habentur. Heidelberg 1681 (2, 4, 13).

716 OLDECOP, MAGN. PET. – Prof. FR. HOFFMANN: De imaginationis natura ejusque viribus. Jena 1687 (7, 9).

717 ORTLOB, ANDREAS: De passione hysterica. Utrecht 1684.

718 ORTLOB, JOH. FRIDERICUS – Prof. BERNHARDUS ALBINUS: De affectibus animi. Frankfurt a. O. 1690 (2, 12).

719 ORTMANN, JOH. CHRISTOPH – Prof. HERMANN PAUL JUCH: De phrenitide. Erfurt 1742 (2, 4, 12).

720 OSCHWALD, JOHANN HENRICUS – Prof. ALBERT HALLER: De phrenitide. Göttingen 1747 (1, 4, 7, 9).

721 OSENBRUCK, GEORG THEODORUS – Prof. ALBERT RUSIL: De suffocatione hypochondriaca et uterina. Leyden 1672 (4, 8, 9, 23).

722 OTTO, JOHANN FRIDR. – Prof. MICHAEL ALBERTI: Animi affectuum medico effectu. Halle 1735 (4).

723 OTTO, JOHANN SEBAST.: De fascinatione puerorum et adultorum. Strasbourg 1664 (4, 16).

724 OTTO, JOHANNES JOSEPHUS – Prof. JOHANN ANDREAS FISCHER: De malo hypochondriaco. Erfurt 1732.

725 OUWENS, WILHELMUS: de horrore. Leyden 1737 (8).

726 OWMAN, MARTINUS – Prof. STEPHAN LE MOYNE: De melancholia. Leyden 1677 (8, 9, 23).

727 PACKBUSCH, STEPHEN. LUDOW.: De progressu morborum spirituum. Leyden 1696 (7, 9, 23).

728 PALTZEL, JOANNES-GEORGIUS: An catalepsi potio cardiaca cathartico emetica? Montpellier 1710 (11).

729 PANECIUS: De ecstasi. Wittenberg 1695.

730 PAPAI, FRANC. PARIZ – Prof. M. ALBERTI: De medicina et doctrina moralis nexu. Halle 1714.

731 PAPEN, CHR. H. – Prof. JO. W. ALBRECHT: De spiritu vini ejusque usu et abusu. Göttingen 1735 (8).

732 PARCOVIUS, FRANCISCUS – Prof. DUNCAN LIDDEL: De melancholia. Helmstadt 1596 (misprint, see no 578).

733 PASOR, MATTH.: De ebrietate. Groningen 1653 (23).

734 PASSELIUS, CASPAR – Prof. JOHANN SPERLING: De magia naturali. Wittenberg 1651 (13).

735 PASTON, IAC.: De phrenitide. Leyden 1584 (8).

736 PAULI, HENRICUS – Prof. WILHELM LAUREN: Propositiones sequentes de melancholia, curatio. Rostock 1593 (9, 17).

737 PAULITZ, JOHANNES THEOD.: De morbis animatis. Leyden 1696 (8).

738 PECK, JOH. CHRISTOPHORUS – Prof. MICHAEL ALBERTI: De phrenitide panoniae idiopathica. Halle 1739 (2, 4, 5).

739 PENZ (PANZ), MICHAEL – Prof. JOHANN JAC. BAIER: De malo hypochondriaco. Altdorf 1709 (9).

740 PERERIUS, BERNARD: An (quaemodum morbi haereditarii) ita et animi mores nobis a parantibus esse possint? Montpellier 1617 (11).

741 PERRELLUS, JACOBUS – Prof. MICHAELE TOUTAIN: An in melancholia divine? Paris 1612 (14).

742 PESTALOZZI, BAPTISTA: De melancholia. Basel 1615 (1, 13).

743 PETRO, JOHANN: De morbis archealibus. Erfurt 1692 (12).

744 PEURSUM, GYSBERTUS VAN: De phrenitide. Utrecht 1711 (18).

745 PFAFF, CHR. M.: De operationibus diabolicis in hoc mundo. Tübingen 1733.

746 PFANKUCH, DANIEL HEINRICH – Prof. JOH. HEINR. FUERSTENAU: De mania. Rinteln 1739 (9, 12).

747 PFEIFFER, HENRICUS GODOFREDUS: De mania. Leyden 1742 (8, 13).

748 PFEIFFER, SIEGMUND AUGUST – Prof. EBERHARD BARNSTOFF: De imperio phanthasmiae in sensu. Greifswald 1707 (9).

749 PFEYL, JOANNES – Prof. HENRICUS STRÖMER: Decreta aliquot medica – Utrum ebrietas vino. Leipzig 1531 (9).

750 PFLAUMB, JOHANNES CHRISTOPHORUS: De phrenitide vera. Leyden 1729 (2, 4, 8).

751 PHILIPPE, JOHAN. DAVID – Prof. JOHAN JACOB HARDER: De catalepsi. Basel 1686 (1, 4, 5, 7, 9).

752 PHILLIPPUS, JOHANNES – Prof. JUSTUS VESTI: De phrenitide. Jena 1692 (5).

753 PIETRE, JOANNES – Prof. GERMANUS PREAUX: An temperamentum melancholicum heroïcum? Paris 1633 (14).

754 PINTO, JOSEPHUS JEZURUN: De phrenitide. Leyden 1694 (8).

755 PISTORIUS, HERMANN – Prof. DUNCAN LIDDEL: De animalis facultate. Helmstadt ca. 1596 (13).

756 PISTORIUS, JOH.: Pentas miscellanea (De vertigine tenebricosa; de melancholia hypochondriaca; de febre quartana; assertiones; problemata). Basel 1605 (1).

757 PISTORIUS, M. GUST. FR.: De existentia spectrorum, et sagarum, veneficorumque pactis cum daemone sancitis. Wittenberg 1703.

758 PIZLER, ANDREA – Prof. GEORG WOLFFGANG WEDEL: De affectibus soporosis et catalepsi ex epitome praexeos clinicae. Jena 1708 (2, 6).

759 PLAATMAN, GERARDUS: De hysterica passione. Utrecht 1724 (18).

760 PLATO, J. J.: De phrenitide. Leyden 1691.

761 PLATTER, FRANZ: De tarantismo. Basel 1669 (1, 10, 13).

762 POIS, CLAUDIUS DE – Prof. JOANNE MERLET: An melancholicis hemorrhoides salutares? Paris 1615 (14).

763 (POLIS, MELCHIOR): De uteri suffocatione. Frankfurt a. O. n.d.

764 POLIS, MELCHIOR – Prof. A. LUDTKE: De affectu hypochondriaco. Frankfurt a. O. 1645 (9).

765 POLLIO, GISB.: De possessione. Leyden 1606.

766 POLNER, ZACHARIAS: De insania. Basel 1632 (5).

767 POSNER, CASPAR: De mania. Jena 1657.

768 POTT, CARL WILHELM – Prof. MICHAEL ALBERTI: De camphorae circumspecto usu medico. Halle 1722 (2).

769 PRETTENUS, JOH. RAPHAEL – Prof. JACOB WOLFF: De cerevisia Numburgensi. Jena 1684 (4, 5).

770 PRINTZ, CAELESTINUS AMANDUS – Prof. GEORG WOLFFGANG WEDEL: De mania. Jena 1708 (4, 6, 12).

771 PROVANSAL, J. A. – Prof. S. P. HILSCHER: De mutuo animae cum corpore commercio et illius cogitatione alte defixa agoniam protrahente. Jena 1744.

772 PUYLON, GILBERTUS – Prof. GUILLELMO DUVAL: An insaniae ab amore? Paris 1630 (14).

773 QUANTEAL, CLAUDE DE – Prof. DOMINIO DE FARCY: Est-ne faemina viro salacior? Paris 1669 (9, 14).

774 QUARTUS, CHR. – Prof. AD. LUCHTENIUS: De melancholia, disp. secunda, in qua de tertia melancholiae specie, quae ex hypochondriis originem ducit, agitur. Helmstadt 1609 (4).

775 QUIQUEBOEUF, CLAUDIUS – Prof. GUILELLMUS DU VAL: An aqua vino salubrior? Paris 1622 (9, 14).

776 QUISTORP, JOHANN BERNHARD – Prof. GEORG DETHARDING: De anaesthesia. Rostock 1718 (2, 4).

777 RABENER, JUSTUS GOTTHART: Disp. I & II. De daemonibus. Leipzig 1706 (7).

778 RABINER, JUSTUS GOTTHART: De daemonibus. Leipzig 1706 (identical with 777).

779 RAESVELT, THOMAS LUDOLF – Prof. HERMANN WITSIUS: De melancholia. Utrecht 1687 (9, 17).

780 RAINSSANT, PIERRE – Prof. FRANCOIS DE LA FRAMBOISIÈRE: An philtris amor conciliari possit? Reims 1649 (15).

781 RAU, JACOB: De malo aphrodiseo. Utrecht 1697.

782 RAUSCHELBACH, JOHANNES ERNESTUS – Prof. W. H. WALDSCHMIDT: De incantantis. Jena 1701 (12, 19).

783 REH, GUILIELMUS: An lac hypochondriacis conveniat? Montpellier 1617 (11).

784 REICH, JOHANN JACOB – Prof. GEORG ERNST STAHL: De passionibus animi corpus humanum. Halle 1695 (2, 4, 5, 12).

785 REICHE, JULIUS – Prof. JOH. DAVID BÜTTNER: De amuletis. Strasbourg 1673.

786 REIN, JOHANNES DAVID – Prof. MARCI MAPPI: De superstitione et remediis superstitionis insignioribus. Strasbourg 1677 (19).

787 REISKE, CHR. HEINR. – Prof. JOHANN ANDREAS FISCHER: De animae vigilii cura corpus humanum. Erfurt 1720 (4).

788 RELOVIUS, CHRISTOPHOR – Prof. JOHANNES ARNOLD FRIDERICI: De affectus hypochondriaci genuina indole. Jena 1662 (6, 12).

789 RENAUDOT, ISAAC – Prof. DIONYSIUS JONCQUET: An insanienti amore virgini venae sectio? Paris 1639 (14).

790 RENAUDOT, EUSEBIUS (ISAAC) – Prof. FLORIMONDUS LANGLOS: An epilepsiae, et melancholiae hemorrhoides salutares? Paris 1640 (14).

791 RENOUARD, LUDOVICUS – Prof. JACOB COUSINOT: An ut corporis, rei animi medicina medetur? Paris 1697 (14).

792 RENTZIUS, GE. – Prof. GE. EHRH. HAMBERGER: De melancholia hypochondriaca s. flatuosa. Tübingen 1595 (4, 17).

793 REVERT, JOANNES BAPTISTA: An melancholicis sit vera confectio alkermes antitodus? Montpellier 1609 (11).

794 RHENANUS, JOHANN – Prof. HENRICUS PETREUS: De melancholia. Marburg 1615 (9).

795 RHODA, FRIDER. WILHELM DE – Prof. RUDOLF WILHELM CRAUSE: De opisthotono. Jena 1696.

796 RHOENIUS, JOHANN – Prof. MICH. ETTMÜLLER: Theses psychologicae. Naturam et essentiam animae duabus definitionibus ab Aristotele descriptam. Leipzig 1699 (2).

797 RICHTER, CHRISTIAN ALBERTUS – Prof. GEORG ERNST STAHL: Qua temperamenta physiologico-physiognomico-pathologico-mechanica. Halle 1697 (2).

798 RICHTER, CH. S. – Prof. G. E. STAHL: De affectibus periodicis. Halle 1702.

799 RICHTER, GEORG GOTTLOB – Prof. WILHELM HULDRICUS WALDSCHMIDT: De mirabili sanatione mulieris Bremensis. Kiel 1726 (13, 17).

800 RIEGER, JOHANNES CHRISTOPHORUS: De anxietate. Leyden 1724 (2, 8).

801 RIEMER, J. E. – Prof. J. A. WEDEL: De affectu hypochondriaco. Jena 1728 (4).

802 RIGIUS, HEINUS: De affectione hypochondriaco. Leyden 1649 (2).

803 ROCAMORA, SAL. DE: De malo aphrodisiaco. Leyden 1738 (7, 8).

804 ROEDER, JOHANN JOSEF: De phrenitide. Altdorf 1644 (4).

805 ROEDER, JOSEF IGNATIUS – Prof. JOANNES FRIDERICUS DE PRÉ: De raro affectu cataleptico. Erfurt 1721 (4, 5, 7).

806 ROEDIGER, JOAN. FRIDERICUS – Prof. JOANNE HENR. SCHULZE: Sitens resolutionem casus hysterico-epileptici. Halle 1736 (4)   .

807 ROESER, CARL AUGUST: De phantasia morborum causa et medicina. Königsberg 1703 (9).

808 ROESER, C. F. – Prof. JACOB FINCKENAU: De phanthasiae efficacia in corpus humanum. Königsberg 1705.

809 ROESER, GEORG HIERONYMUS: De philtrorum agendi modo et noxis. Altdorf 1701.

810 RÖSER, JOHANNES – Prof. JOHANN GERHARD WINTHER: De Admirando illo Affectu Catalepsi. Rinteln 1692.

811 ROGERS, JOSEPHUS: De affectione hysterica. seu hypochondriaca. Utrecht 1708 (18).

812 ROMELIUS, THEOD. REN. – Prof. GEORG WOLFFGANG WEDEL: De amorum natura et usu. Jena 1692 (4).

813 RONTRIS, CASPAR: De hysterica passione. Utrecht 1674.

814 ROTH, SEBAST. – Prof. ANTON VARUS: De melancholia desipientia. Jena 1610 (12).

815 ROTHMANN, JOH.: De morborum causis ex coeli ac siderum influxu. Basel 1592 (1).

816 ROTTENBERGER, JOHANN – Prof. GEORG WOLFGANG WEDEL: De acta Literatorum. Erfurt 1674 (2).

817 RUEDIGER JOHANNES LUDOVICUS – Prof. JOH. JUNKER: De variabili hypochondriacorum mente. Halle 1746 (6, 7, 12).

818 RUGENWALD, JOANNES – Prof. JOH. GOTTFR. BERGER: De errore diaetae in potu. Wittenberg 1709 (6, 12, 13).

819 RUOFF, CHRISTOPH: De melancholiae natura, causis et differentiis. Strasbourg 1626 (4).

820 RUPERTUS, CHRISTOPH HENRICUS: De malo hypochondriaco. Erfurt 1674.

821 RUPERTUS, JACOBUS THOMAS: De hysterica passione. Utrecht 1724 (18).

822 RUPITZ, ARET. – Prof. P. AMAN: De affectione hypochondriaca. Leipzig 1666.

823 RUPITZ, VALENTINUS: De praefocatione hysterica. Leipzig 1623 (2).

824 RUROCK, JOHANNES CHRISTIANUS – Prof. CAROLUS DRELINCURTIUS: De passione hysterica. Leyden 1679 (8).

825 RUSSIUS: De passione hysterica. Leyden 1692 (8) (see BUSSIUS).

826 RUTTORFER, JOHANNES JEREMIAS – Prof. JOHANN THEODOR SCHENCK: De phrenitide. Jena 1666 (4, 5).

827 RYHINER, JOH. HEINR. – Prof. JOH. NIC. STUPANUS: De animae humanae facultatibus, functionibus ac sedibus. Basel 1598 (1).

828 SACHS, ESAIAS – Prof. DUNCAN LIDDEL: De sensibus interioribus, de facultate principe secundum medicos, de facultate intellectua et locomotoria. Helmstadt 1597 (13a).

829 SACK, ERASMUS – Prof. JACOB GOLIUS: De minera et medela affectionis hypochondriacae, ... affectionis scorbuticae et hystericae dictae. Leyden 1665 (8).

830 SALMUTH, JOHANNES HEINRICUS – Prof. ERNESTUS HENRICUS WEDEL: De morbis concionatorum. Jena 1699 (4, 6, 9, 17).

831 (SALZMANN, JOHANN RUDOLPH): De mania ejusque speciebus lycanthropia et hydrophobia. Strasbourg 1619 (16).

832 (SALZMANN, JOHANN RUDOLPH): De phrenitide. Strasbourg 1637 (4).

833 SANCHE, PETRUS: An electuarium diaphaeniconis hystericis affectibus conveniat? Montpellier 1619 (11).

834 SANDIUS, JOH.: De possessione. Leyden 1597 (8).

835 SAUTYN, ELIAS – Prof. THEOD. CRAANEN: De mania. Leyden 1676.

836 SCHAABNER, A. J. W.: De phrenitide. Prague 1744.

837 SCHAAR, GEORG – Prof. GUILIELMUS BAIER: De phantasia matre enthusiasmi. Altdorf 1721 (9).

838 SCHACHER, P.: De melancholia hypochondriaca. Leipzig 1732.

839 SCHACHT, HERMANN OOSTERDYCK: De melancholia hypochondriaca. Leyden 1693 (2, 4, 8, 23).

840 SCHACHT, HERM. OOSTERDYCK: Disputatio philosophica inauguralis, de sensibus internis memoria et imaginatione. Leyden 1693 (8, 9).

841 SCHAEFFER, JOHANN CHRISTIAN – Prof. CHRISTIAN VATER: Solemnen de morbo sontico sacro. Wittenberg 1702 (6).

842 SCHAEFFER, LUDOLPH – Prof. GEORG DETHARDING: Specimen manuductionis ad vitam longam quod tradit regulas generales, circa animi affectus hominibus observandas. Wie überhaupt in Beobachtung der Gemühts Bewegungen der Mensch sein Leben höher bringen könne. Rostock 1724 (2, 4).

843 SCHAEVIUS, – Prof. WERNER ROLFINCK: De phrenitide. Jena 1650 (13a).

844 SCHÄRF, Io. A.: De phrenitide. Altdorf 1746 (4, 12).

845 SCHAPER, JOHANNES ERNESTUS: De malo hysterico in viris. Rostock 1699 (24).

846 SCHAW, GULIELMUS – Prof. JACOBUS SMITH: De morbis ex animi passionibus orientibus. Edinburgh 1735 (2).

847 SCHEER: De melancholia hypochondriaca. Giessen 1677.

848 SCHEFFER, SEBASTIAN – Prof. JACOB TAPPIUS: De melancholica desipientia. Helmstadt 1652 (5).

849 SCHEFFLER, CHRISTIAN JOANNES – Prof. CONRAD JOHRENIUS: Idolum muliebre in vulgò ita dietâ passione hysterica. Frankfurt a. O. 1707 (4, 6).

850 SCHEID, JOHANN GOTTFRIED: Brevis historiae mulieris cuiusdam, quae inopinato casu subito loquelam amisit, et ex insperato repente recepit, enodatio. Strasbourg 1725 (16, 20).

851 SCHENCK, JOHANN THEODOR – Prof. W. ROLFINCK: De melancholia hypochondriaca. Jena 1644 (4, 7, 10, 13a, 17).

852 SCHIFFMAN, THOMAS – Prof. ISRAEL SPACH: De animi affectibus. Strasbourg 1598 (2).

853 SCHIFFMANN, THOM.: De hysterica affectione. Basel 1600 (1, 13).

854 SCHILLER, JO. GOTTL. – Prof. CHR. GOD. STENTZEL: Morbos corporis morbis mentis non curari nec curandos esse demonstrat. Wittenberg 1736 (19).

855 SCHILLING, JOHANNES: Aegrum ex amore catalepticum factum proponens. Giessen 1676 (2, 4, 5, 9, 13).

856 SCHLAPPERITIUS, JOHANN LUDWIG – Prof. GEORG WOLFGANG WEDEL: De mania. Jena 1673 (5, 6).

857 SCHLEICH, JO. LEONH.: De passione hysterica. Leyden 1675 (8).

858 SCHLEIERMACHER, GEORG LUDWIG: De catalepsi, rarissimo affectuum. Giessen 1695 (5).

859 SCHMID, ZACHARIAS GOTTFRIED – Prof. MICHAEL ALBERTI: De mente sana in corpore sano. Halle 1728 (2, 5, 9, 12, 19).

860 SCHMIDIUS, JUSTUS ANDREAS – Prof. AUGUSTINUS HENRICUS FASCH: De suffocatione uterino. Jena 1681 (4, 5).

861 SCHMIDER, SIG. – Prof. CH. L. WELSCH: De superstitiosa morborum cura christiano atque dogmatico medico indigna. Leipzig 1710.

862 SCHMIDT, AUG. JO. – Prof. TH. LUTHER: De malo hypochondriaco. Erfurt 1737 (7).

863 SCHMIDT, CHRISTOPHORUS PHILIPPUS – Prof. GEORG ERNEST STAHL: De animi morbis. Halle 1708 (5, 7, 9, 12).

864 SCHMIDT, PAUL – Prof. J. RUDOLPH SALZMANN: De melancholia hypochondriaca. Strasbourg 1621 (4).

865 SCHMILAUER, PETER – Prof. TOBIAS TANDLER: De melancholia natura, causis, differentitis & signis. Wittenberg 1608 (10, 13a).

866 SCHMILAUER, PETER: De melancholiorum divinatione. Wittenberg 1608 (10, 13).

867 SCHMITNER, ASSVERUS (AHASVERUS) – Prof. CASPAR BAUHIN: De phrenitide. Basel 1612 (1, 6, 13).

868 SCHNEIDER, JOHANN CCHRISTIAN – Prof. JO. PH. EYSEL: De scandalis medicorum. Erfurt 1716 (5).

869 SCHOLTE, JOHANNES FRANCISCUS: De passione hysterica seu suffocatione hypochondriaca. Utrecht 1730 (13).

870 SCHOLTETUS, HIEREMIA – Prof. DUNCAN LIDDEL: De causis symptomatum motus voluntarii. Helmstadt 1598 (13a).

871 SCHOMBURG, JOHANN – Prof. GEORG WOLFFGANG WEDEL: De catalepsi rarissimo affectuum. Jena 1690 (4, 6).

872 SCHOMBURG, JOSIA SIGM. – Prof. GEORG WOLFFGANG WEDEL: De strangulatione uteri syncoptica laborans. Jena 1717.

873 SCHONWALDER, MELCHIOR – Prof. GREGOR HORST: De poculis amatoriis. Giessen 1611 (13a).

874 SCHOOKIUS, MART.: De exstasi. Groningen 1661 (23).

875 SCHÖTTEL, FRIDR. – Prof. NIC. AGERIUS: De anima. Strasbourg 1622.

876 SCHOUTEN, DIRK: De anxietata. Leyden 1742 (8).

877 SCHRAGE, JOHANNES: De melancholia. Leyden 1695 (8, 10).

878 SCHREINER, GEORG EBERHARD – Prof. JOHANN GERHARD: De amore insano ejusque cura. Tübingen 1633 (17).

879 SCHROEDER, CASPAR HENRICUS – Prof. ERNST GOTTHOLD STRUVE: Ideam mali hypochondriaci ejusque praeservationem. Kiel 1741 (17).

880 SCHRÖDER, FRANZ: De phrenitide. Basel 1584 (1).

881 SCHRÖDER, (SCHROEER?), JOH. FRID. – Prof. JOHANN PHILIPP EYSEL: Aegrum affectu maniaco laborantem sistens. Erfurt 1695 (4, 5, 10).

882 SCHROETER, PAUL – Prof. MARC. BANZER: De melancholia hypochondriaca. Wittenberg 1645 (7, 10).

883 SCHROETER, P. D.: De catalepsi. Utrecht 1692 (4, 9).

884 SCHUBART, F. C.: De potentia diaboli in sensus hominum. Jena 1746.

885 SCHULTETUS, CASP.: De phrenitide. Basel 1593 (1).

886 SCHULTZ, GOTHOFREDUS – Prof. IRENAEUS VEHR: De melancholia ex utero, in puerperâ observatâ & curatâ. Frankfurt a. O. 1705 (2, 5, 12, 17).

887 SCHULTZ, JEREMIAH – Prof. SAMUEL POMARIUS: De noctambulis. Disputatio posterior. Wittenberg 1650 (6, 12).

888 SCHULZ, ZACHARIAS PHILIPPUS – Prof. MICHAEL ALBERTI: De euthanasia medica. Halle 1735 (4).

889 SCHUR, J. THEOD.: De melancholia hypochondriaca. Giessen 1677 (4).

890 SCHURER, HENNING – Prof. CHRISTIAN LANGE: De memoria. Leipzig 1650.

891 SCHWANSHOFER, MICHAEL – Prof. ZACHARIAS BRENDEL: De affectu hypochondriaco. Jena 1637 (5).

892 SCHWARTZ, CHR. G. – Prof. BÜCHNER, ANDREAS ELIAS VON: De genuinis opii effectibus in corpore humano. Halle 1748.

893 SCHWARTZ, WILHELMUS HEINRICUS – Prof. WERNER ROLFINCK: De lienis, affectu hypochondriaco et scorbutus. Jena (13a).

894 SCHWEITZER, CHR.: De passione hysterica. Leyden 1684 (1, 10).

895 SCHWENCKFELT, CASP.: De melancholia. Basel 1587 (1).

896 SCHWIMMER, JOH. MICH.: De spectris. Halle 1689.

897 SCLANCFIUS, HECTOR: Quaestiones hasce Medicas publicè examinandas proponit. Marburg 1601 (2).

898 (SEBIZ, MELCH.): De affectione hypochondriaca. Strasbourg 1682 (4).

899 SEELIGER, CHRISTOPHORUS: De suffocatione uteri. Leyden 1662 (8, 10).

900 SEELMANN, JOH. GOTTLIEB – Prof. BRANDANUS MEIBOM: De animae ad restituendam sanitatem impotentia. Helmstadt 1719 (2).

901 SELPERT, G. A. DE – Prof. GE. GOTTLOB RICHTER: De medicina plagosa. Göttingen 1746.

902 SEMBDER, CHRISTIAN BENJAMIN – Prof. CHRISTIAN MICHAEL ADOLPHI.: De affectu mirachiali. Leipzig 1734 (5, 9).

903 SENNERT, MICHAEL: De affectione hypochondriaca. Wittenberg 1628 (6).

904 SERON, ANDREAS JOSEPHUS – Prof. FRANCISCUS AIGNAN: An ab animi pathematis functionum laesio? Paris 1721 (14).

905 SEUFFERHELD, GUIL. NIC.: De morbis bibonum. Altdorf 1720.

906 's GRAVESANDE, GUILIELMUS JACOBUS: De autocheiria. Leyden 1707 (8).

907 SHERWOOD, RICHARDUS: De morbis a potus spirituosi abusu oriundis. Leyden
1739 (8).

908 SIBER, JOH. GE. – Prof. GEORG WOLFFGANG WEDEL: De terrorum natura, usu
et abusu. Jena 1697 (4–6).

909 SIFERT, ADAM – Prof. DUNCAN LIDDEL: De symptomatibus et symptomatum
differentiis. Helmstadt 1598 (13a).

910 SINAPIUS, MICHAEL ALOYSIUS – Prof. AUG. HENR. FASCH: De mania. Jena
1701 (5).

911 SIRET, RENATUS: An phrenitidi balneum? Montpellier 1710 (11).

912 SISMUS, CORNELIUS: De suffocatione stomachia. Leyden 1695 (8).

913 (SLEGEL, PAUL MARQUARD): De affectione hypochondriaca. Jena 1641.

914 SNOECK, GERARDUS: De mania. Utrecht 1671 (5, 18).

915 SOLINUS, JOHANNES: De melancholia. Utrecht 1678.

916 SOMMER, HENRICUS GOTHOFREDUS – Prof. GEORG WOLFFGANG WEDEL: De
mania. Jena 1693 (4, 5).

917 SOMMER, JOANNES CASPARUS: De melancholia imprimis hypochondriaca. Leyden 1706 (8).

918 SOMMERFELDT, IO. GOTTLIEB – Prof. JOH. ADOLF WEDEL: De deliriis in genere. Jena 1744 (2, 4, 6).

919 SONDEN, JO. HENR. VON – Prof. FRIDERICH HOFFMANN: Sistens affectum spas-
modico-hypochondriacum inveteratum. Halle 1734.

920 SONER, ERNST: De melancholia. Basel 1601 (1, 13).

921 SPERLING, JO.: De magia naturali et demoniaca. Wittenberg 1630.

922 (SPERLING, JO.): De viribus imaginationis. Wittenberg 1639.

923 (SPERLING, JO.): De spectris. Wittenberg 1649.

924 SPIESS, JOHANNES HENRICUS – Prof. JUSTUS VESTI: De magnetismus marcro- et
microcosmi. Erfurt 1695 (2, 5).

925 (STAHL, IVO): De passione hysterica. Erfurt 1729.

926 (STAHL, IVO): De malo hypochondriaco. Erfurt 1739.

927 STAMPERIUS, JOHANNES: De melancholia. Utrecht 1668.

928 STANGIUS, JOHANN JACOB – Prof. FRIDERICUS HOFFMANN: De mentis morbis,
ex morbosa sanguinis circulatione ortis. Halle 1700 (2, 5, 7, 12).

929 STANGIUS, SAMUEL – Prof. TOBIAS KNOBLOCHIUS: De partibus continentibus
capits. Wittenberg 1622 (13a).

930 STARCKE, HEINRICH – Prof. JOACHIM STOCKMANN: De somno, nyktegersia ecstasi et ephialte. Rostock 1625.

931 STEGMANN, JOHANNES JOSUA – Prof. MICHAEL ALBERTI: De abstinentia medici
ab aegrotis famam et vitam nonnunquam conservante. Greifswald 1722 (2).

932 STEGMAYERUS, JOH. GEORGIUS: De furore hysterico, vel uterino. Altdorf 1713
(2, 4, 5, 17, 20).

933 STEIGELL, J. G.: De mania. Rinteln 1725.

934 STEIGERTHAL, JOHANN GEORG – Prof. FRIDERICUS SCHRADER: De imaginationis
maternae in foetum efficacia. Helmstadt 1686 (9).

935 STEIN – Prof. ZACH. BRENDEL: De melancholia. Jena 1618 (4, 17).

936 STEINBACH, M. J.: De phrenitide. 1740.

937 STEINER, HULDR.: De anxietate. Basel 1739 (1).

938 STEININGER, JOAN. ALBERTUS – Prof. MAURICIUS BLUM: De melancholia hypochondriaca. Wittenberg 1625 (1).

939 STEPHANI, JOH. JAC.: De somnambulis. Basel 1701 (1).

940 STERNBECK, VALENTIUS PAULUS – Prof. JUSTUS VESTI: De affectione hypochondriaca. Erfurt 1702 (6, 7, 12).

941 STERNBERG, CHRISTOPHORUS: De suffocatione uteri. Leyden 1652 (2, 5, 9).

942 STEVER, CHRISTIAN FRIDERICH – Prof. GEORG DETHARDINGIUS: De obsessione eademque spuria, von besessenen und von besessen gehaltenen Menschen. Rostock 1721 (7, 9, 17, 19).

943 STIRNA, JAC. – Prof. J. J. WALDSCHMIDT: Physicae curiosae et utilis specimen de sensibus. Marburg 1686 (13).

944 STOCHIUS, ANTONIUS: De affectione hypochondriaca. Utrecht 1730 (2).

945 STOCKE, LEONARDUS – Prof. JOHANNES OOSTENDYK SCHACHT: De terrore ejusque effectis in corpus humanum. Utrecht 1733 (18).

946 STOCKMANN, JOACHIM – Prof. JACOB FABRICIUS: De deliriis in venere et in specie de phrenitide. Rostock 1619 (24).

947 STOCKMANN, JO. CAR. – Prof. ANDR. EL. BUECHNER: De variae therapiae necessitate tam in hypochondriaco quam hysterico malo. Halle 1747 (13).

948 STOLL, JOHANNES – Prof. HENRICUS PETRAEUS: De suffocatione & procidentia uteri. Marburg 1616 (9).

949 STOLLE, FRIDERICUS HENRICUS: De phrenitide idiopathica. Leyden 1733 (2, 4, 8, 9).

950 STOLTERFOHT, JOH. JAC. – Prof. JOHANN GERDESIUS: Ideam errantem in ecstasi seu enthusiasmo conspicuam. Greifswald 1692 (2, 4, 19).

951 STOLTZEN, JOHANNE GOTTLIEB – Prof. G. CASP. KIRCHMAIER: De apparitionibus spectror. & spirituum. Wittenberg 1692 (4, 17).

952 STORCK, JOHANNES CHRISTOPHORUS: De malo hypochondriaco. Altdorf 1685 (7, 9).

953 STORMIUS, JANUS PETRUS – Prof. ANSAGARIUS ANCHERSON: De medicatione per musicam. (Diss. primo) Copenhagen 1720 (2, 21).

954 STRASSBURG, JOH. GEORG: De melancholia hypochondriaca. Basel 1650 (1, 17, 24).

955 STRASBURG, JOH. THEOD. – Prof. ADAM HARWECK: De affectu hypochondriaco. Königsberg 1696.

956 STRAUSS, JOHANN DANIEL: Aegrum affectu hypochondriaco. Giessen 1683 (12).

957 STRAUSS, LAURENTIUS – Prof. WERNER ROLFINCK: De melancholia. Jena 1635 (13a).

958 STRUVE, CAROLUS GUILIELMUS FRIDERICUS – Prof. GTTL. HENR. KANNEGIESSER: De spiritu ardente ejusque modo operandi disquisitio. Kiel 1747 (17).

959 STRUVE, ERNST GOTTHOLD – Prof. G. E. STAHL: De facie morborum indice seu morborum aestimatione ex facie. Halle 1700 (19).

960 STRUVE, JOHANNES ADAMUS – Prof. MICHAEL ALBERTI: De spectris. Halle 1725 (2, 5, 9).

961 STRUYCKMAN, GERARDUS: De melancholia hypochondriaca. Utrecht 1694 (18).

962 STRYKIUS: De dementia et melancholia. Frankfurt a. O. 1683.

963 STUBENDORF, JOS. – Prof. VAL. ESPICH: De melancholia. Wittenberg 1585 (4).

964 SUCHTELEN, PETRUS VAN – Prof. JOHANN JACOB RAU: De melancholia hypochondriaca. Leyden 1718 (2, 4, 8).

965 SUESS, JOHANNES PHILIPPUS – Prof. JACOB SCHALLER: De sobrietate. Strasbourg 1656 (2).

966 SUPPRIAN, FRIDER. LEBERECHT – Prof. IO. GOTTLIEB KRUGER: De physiognomiae in re medica utilitate. Greifswald 1745 (2).

967 SÜSSENBACH, CHRISTOPHORUS – Prof. MICHAEL ALBERTI: De Therapia imaginaria. Von Menschen die aus Einbildung gesund werden. Halle 1721 (13, 17).

968 TACKIUS, EBERHARD: De nostalgia. Giessen 1707.

969 TESSARARIUS, JEREMIA – Prof. VALERIUS CHARSTADIUS: De animae facultatibus et earum functionibus. Strasbourg 1626 (2, 16).

970 TEUTSCHER, JO. CHRISTIAN – Prof. JOANNES FRIDERICUS DE PRÉ: De usu et abusu amuletorum – Von Brauch und Misbrauch der Anhängsel wider die Kranckheiten. Erfurt 1720 (2, 5, 7).

971 THEIL (THEILL), LAURENTIUS – Prof. JOH. THEOD. SCHENCK: De malo hypochondriaco. Jena 1668 (12).

972 THEISNER, JOHANN JACOB – Prof. JOHANN THEODOR SCHENCK: De ambulatione in somno. Jena 1671 (6).

973 THEVART, ABR. – Prof. DIONYSIUS GUERIN: Est melancholicis brevioris vitae? Paris 1655 (14).

974 THIEBOUT, THEODORUS: De phrenitide. Utrecht 1674.

975 THIEME, JOHANN PHILIPP – Prof. JUSTUS VESTI: De phrenitide. Erfurt 1692 (4, 5).

976 THIEPHAINE, FRANCISCUS – Prof. AEGIDIUS CULOTEAU: An temperamentum melancholicum praestantius? Reims 1704 (15).

977 THILEN, JO.: De analepsi rationali (including Vater, Abraham-pro. de animae et corporis commercio). Wittenberg 1727.

978 THILO, JOH. FR. – Prof. JOH. ANDR. FISCHER: De convulsionibus epilepticis habitualibus ex terrore. Erfurt 1727 (4, 7).

979 THOCQUESNE, ANTOINE – Prof. FRANÇOIS DE LA FRAMBOISIÈRE (author?): An Phrenitidi phlebotomia et catharsis? Reims 1656 (15).

980 THOMÉ, ST.: An somnambulis balneum? Avignon 1713.

981 THONER, AUG.: De melancholia. Basel 1590 (1, 13).

982 THUILLIER, CHARLES – Prof. RENATO LE CONTE: An cerevisia, potus saluberrimus? Paris 1695 (14).

983 TILEMAN genannt SCHENCK, ADOLPHUS – Prof. STEPHANI LE MOYNE: De epilepsia hypochondriaca. Leyden 1677 (8, 9).

984 TILING, JOHANNIS: De suffocatione hypochondriaco. Leyden 1692 (4, 8).

985 TITIUS, CHR. – Prof. JO. HADR. SLEVOGT: De autochiria medica in genere. Jena 1707.

986 TITSCHARDO, GEORGIUS – Prof. GREGOR HORST: De causis symptomatum facultatis motivae principis (9, 13a).

987 TROESTER, CHRISTIAN ANDREAS – Prof. JOHANN ADOLPH WEDEL: Sistens aegrum melancholia hypochondriaca laborantem. Jena 1717 (2, 4, 5, 12).

988 TROPPENNIGER, JOH. CHRIST. – Prof. MICH. ETTMÜLLER: De malo hypochondriaco. Leipzig 1676 (2).

989 TROTZ, CHRISTIAN: De deliriis. Strasbourg 1740 (12).

990 TSCHIMESIUS, FRID. – Prof. J. RUDOLPH SALZMANN: De phrenitide et paraphrenitide. Strasbourg 1617 (4).

991 UNVERZAGT, HENNINGUS – Prof. JOANNE WOLFIUS: De melancholia. Helmstadt 1614 (9).

992 UNSENIUS, JOHANNES – Prof. ECCARD LEICHNER: De hysteromania. Erfurt 1671 (5).

993 UMBGROVE, LUBBERTUS: De phrenitide vera. Leyden 1717 (4, 8).

994 VALCKENAAR, ABRAHAM: De animi affectionibus. Leyden 1748 (8, 19).

995 VARIN, ANTONIUS – Prof. JOANNES ANTONIUS BOURGAUD: An in morbis melancholicis purgatio per inferiora? Paris 1685 (14).

996 (VARUS, ANTON): De mania et desipientia. Jena 1606.

997 VASLET, RAYMUNDUS – Prof. M. CLAUDIUS GERMAIN: An Veternus Delirio Capitalior? Paris 1667 (9, 14).

998 VASSE, DAVID – Prof. LUDOVICUS-SIMONE EMMEREZ: An à mente sanitatis? Paris 1721 (14).

999 VATER, CHRISTIAN – Prof. CONRAD VICTOR SCHNEIDER: De melancholia seu delirio tristi. Wittenberg 1680 (4, 5, 7, 9, 13).

1000 VENATOR, ADOLPH: De melancholia. Leyden 1618 (2, 8).

1001 VENTALO, IGNATIUS: An maniae balnea aquae dulcis? Montpellier 1711 (11).

1002 VERMEIREN, NICOLAUS: De suffocatione hypochondriaca. Leyden 1668 (4, 7, 8).

1003 VERNON, THOMAS: De passione hypochondriaca, hysteria dicta. Leyden 1704 (8, 9).

1004 VESTI, JUSTUS: De malo hypochondriaco. Erfurt 1691.

1005 (VESTI, JUSTUS): Aeger melancholia amatoria variisque symptomatibus gravioribus macitatus. Erfurt 1701.

1006 VIGNE, NIC. DE – Prof. JACOB GAMARRE: Non est fascinum coitum impedit. Paris 1649 (14).

1007 VILELLA, CASIMIRUS: De phrenitide. Leyden 1717 (4, 8).

1008 VISCHER, JOHANN CHRISTIAN – Prof. JO. GOTTHARD TEUTSCHER: De philtris. Leipzig 1711 (2).

1009 VISCHER, J. DE: De phrenitide. Leyden 1676 (9).

1010 VLASBLOM, LUDOVICUS: De melancholia. Utrecht 1663.

1011 VOGEL, JOHANNIS GEORGIUS – Prof. JOANN. ADAM MORASCH: De affectibus paraphoricis seu deliriis. Ingolstadt n.d. (2).

1012 VOGEL, R. L.: De insania. Göttingen 1736.

1013 VOGEL, ST. SIEGR. – Prof. MICHAEL ALBERTI: De spirituum ardentium usu et abusu diaetetico. Halle 1732.

1014 VOGELIUS, TOBIAS – Prof. JOH. ARNOLD FRIDERICI: De memoriae laestione seu oblivione. Jena 1668 (12).

1015 VOGTHER, CONRADUS BUKARDEUS: De morbis moerentium. Altdorf 1703 (2, 12, 17).

1016 VOIGT, JOANNES CASPARUS IGNATIUS: De passione seu affectione hypochondriaca. Tractatus medica. Prague 1678 (2, 13).

1017 VOLLHARDT, JOHAN. JEREMIAS: De melancholia. Strasbourg 1654 (2, 4, 12).

1018 WACHTEL, G. W.: De affectibus animi in genere. Jena 1705.

1019 WACHTEL, JOANNES CHRISTOPH. – Prof. AUGUST HENRICUS FASCH: Exhibens mulierem melancholia hypochondriaca laborantem. Jena 1674 (4, 5, 9, 12).

1020 WALDSCHMIDT, JOHANN JAKOB: De affectione hypochondriaca. Giessen 1666 (7, 13a).

1021 (WALDSCHMIDT, JOHANN JAKOB): De phrenitide, melancholia, mania et hydrophobia. Marburg n.d. (9, 13a).

1022 WALDSCHMIDT, WILHELM HULDERICUS – Prof. JOHANN JACOB WALDSCHMIDT: De morbis Aulicis. Marburg, ca. 1690 (13).

1023 WALLERIUS, HAR.: De fallaciis visionis. Upsula 1703.

1024 WALLICH, GEORG. TOBIAS – Prof. JO. ARN. FRIDERICUS: De mania ex philtro. Jena 1670 (12).

1025 WALLICH, SIMON – Prof. ANTONIUS MATTHAEUS: De melancholia hypochondriaca. Leyden 1678 (4, 8).

1026 WALTERUS, GODOFREDUS: De suffocatione hypochondriaca in viro. Leyden 1688 (2, 4, 8).

1027 WALTHER, AUG. FRIEDRICH: De temperamentis et deliriis. Leipzig 1741.

1028 WALTHER, JOH. – Prof. DUNCAN LIDDEL: De febribus continens putridarum febrium et putredinis, naturam, differentias & causes. Helmstadt 1602 (13a).

1029 WALTHER, GOTTFRIED – Prof. WERNER ROLFINCK: De malancholia. Jena 1652 (13a).

1030 WARDENBURG, JO. HENR. – Prof. MICHAEL ALBERTI: De morbis animi ex anomaliis haemorrhagicis. Halle 1719 (4, 5, 7, 9).

1031 WAXMANN, SIGISMUND – Prof. AUGUST HEINRICH FASCH: De suffocatione hysterica. Jena 1687 (4, 5, 9, 10, 19).

1032 WEBERSKI, JOANNES-JACOBUS: An in phrenitide repellentia? An hystericis castoreum? Montpellier 1682 (11).

1033 WEDEL, ERNST HEINRICH – Prof. GEORG WOLFFGANG WEDEL: De spectris. Jena 1693 (4, 5, 6, 9).

1034 (WEDEL, GEORG W.): De uteri suffocatione. Jena 1674 (4, 6).

1035 WEDEL, JOHANN ADOLPH – Prof. GEORG WOLFFGANG WEDEL: De camphoro. Jena 1697 (5).

1036 WEDIG, J. HIER. DE – Prof. ABR. VATER: De memoria, prasesertim labili. Wittenberg 1691.

1037 WEGENER, ADAMUS – Prof. MICHAEL ALBERTI: De morbis faeminarum virilibus. Halle 1738 (2).

1038 WEIDLER, FRANCISC. EHRENFR. – Prof. JACOB WOLF: De literatorum potu, ejusque usu et abusu. Jena 1684 (4).

1039 WEIGEL, BL. NIC. – Prof. CHR. STEPH. SCHEFFEL: De malo hypochondriaco. Greifswald 1745 (6).

1040 WEINLIN, GEORG NICOLAUS – Prof. ELIAS RUDOLF CAMERARIUS: De phrenitide. Tübingen 1684 (1, 4, 9, 10, 12, 17).

1041 WEISSER, G.: De autocheiria. Giessen 1668.

1042 WEITZ, JACOB: De passione hysterica. Utrecht 1665 (5).

1043 WEITZIUS, HENRIC. SIGISM. – Prof. PAUL GOTTFRIED SPERLING: De deliriis febrium continuarum. Wittenberg 1696 (4, 9, 12).

1044 WELSCH, JOHANN MELCHIOR – Prof. FRIDERICH HOFFMANN: De vini Hungarici Excellente natura, virtute et usu. Halle 1721 (2).

1045 WELTZ, JOHANNES FRANCISCUS – Prof. MICHAEL ALBERTI: De medici officio circa animan in causa sanitatis: Ob die Medizin in Curen mit der Seele etwas zu schaffen habe? Halle 1745 (7, 17).

1046 WEHRT, VAN DER: De catalepsi. Duisburg 1734.

1047 WENDIUS, JOH. CHRISTIAN – Prof. JUSTUS VESTI: De catalepsi. Erfurt 1689 (5, 6, 10, 12).

1048 WENDT, GE. GTTF. – Prof. MICHAEL ALBERTI: De anima nec cogitante nec volente, corpus suum internum movente. Halle 1744.

1049 WERKE, MICHAEL VAN DE: De Paraphrenitide. Leyden 1735 (8).

1050 WERNER, PHILIPPUS – Prof. SIMON OPSOPAEUS: De phrenitide. Heidelberg 1614 (2).

1051 WESLINGH, JOANNES – Prof. CAROL. DRELINCURTIUS: De passione hysterica. Leyden 1694 (17, 19).

1052 WESTENBERG, JOH.: De melancholia. Basel 1618 (1, 13).

1053 WESTHOFF, RUGERUS: De affectu hypochondriaco. Strasbourg 1668 (2).

1054 WILHELM, GOTHOFREDUS ERNESTUS – Prof. JUSTUS VESTI: Sistens aegrum melancholia hypochondriaca laborantem. Erfurt 1704 (4, 5, 12).

1055 WILLI (WILLIUS), JAHANN VALENTIN: Affectum vehementissimum usu, vehementissimorum affectum effectum et causam ira. Strasbourg 1671 (12, 16).

1056 WIND, TOBIAS: De melancholico delirio. Basel 1596 (1).

1057 WINTER, FRIDERICUS – Prof. LUDWIG FRIEDRICH JACOB: De mania. Erfurt 1710 (4, 5, 12).

1058 WIPACHER, DAVID – Prof. JOHANNIS BOHN: Disp. qua casus aegri, somnambulationis morbo laborantis, resolutus sistitur. Leipzig 1717 (4, 13).

1059 WIRSNIZER, GEORG ANTON – Prof. JO. JA. JANTKE: De memoriae laesione. Altdorf 1735 (4).

1060 WIRTHIUS, GALLUS: De affectu hypochondriaco. Basel 1661 (1).

1061 WITT, JOHANNES MICHAEL: De obsessis falsis atque varis. Erfurt 1739 (12, 19).

1062 WITTEN, ALEXANDER – Prof. H. OOSTERDYK SCHACHT: De hysterica passione. Leyden 1722 (2, 8).

1063 WITTICHIUS, NICOLAUS – Prof. JOH. MARTIN JOHRENIUS: De sede animae rationalis. Marburg 1673 (2).

1064 WIZLEBEN: De autocheiria. Leipzig 1702.

1065 WOLF, CHRIST. – Prof. CHR. WANTSCHER: De lupo et lycanthropia. Wittenberg 1666.

1066 WOLF, HENRICUS – Prof. DUNCAN LIDDEL: De febribus continens curationem omnium febrium putridarum in specie. Helmstadt 1620? (13a).

1067 WOLF, JO. GEORG – Prof. HENRICUS CLAUSING: De mentis humanae morbis gravissimis. Wittenberg 1708 (13).

1068 WOLFF, GEORG CONRAD – Prof. BERNHARD ALBINUS: De melancholia. Frankfurt a. O. 1687 (2, 4, 5, 10, 17).

1069 WOLFF, CHRISTIAN JUSTINUS – Prof. RUDOLF WILHELM CRAUSIUS: De memoria ejusque remediorum natura, usu, et abusu. Jena 1696 (4, 6, 9, 10).

1070 WOLFF, JOH.: De phrenitide exquisita. Strasbourg 1633.

1071 WOLFF, JOHANNES CHRISTIAN – Prof. GEORG WOLFFGANG WEDEL: De morbo spasmodico epidemico maligno in Saxonia, Lusatia, vicinisque locis. Jena 1717 (4).

1072 WOLFF, JOHANNES FRIDERICUS – Prof. CHRISTIAN GODOFR. STENTZEL: De philtris rite de examinandis et dividicandis; Von Liebes-Träncken. Wittenberg 1726 (2, 4).

1073 WOLFHARD, LEO – Prof. THOMAS ERASTUS: De melancholia. Basel 1577 (1, 4, 6, 13).

1074 WOLFHARD, MARC. – Prof. JOH. NIC. STUPANUS: De suffocatione appellata hysterica. Basel 1604 (1, 13).

1075 WOLLINIUS, JOHANNES – Prof. JACOB TAPPIUS: De amore insano. Helmstadt 1661 (5).

1076 WOLPHART, CHRISTOPHER JOACHIM: De mania. Basel 1666 (1).

1077 WYCKERSLOOT, JOANNES – Prof. ISBRAND DE DIEMERBROECK: De phrenitide. Utrecht 1650.

1078 WYMPERSSE, JACOBUS THIENSIUS VAN DE: De phrenitide. Leyden 1713 (12, 18).

1079 YON, DURANDUS FRANCISCUS – Prof. FRANCISCUS LE VIGNON: Mutat-ne amor ingenium? Paris 1635 (14).

1080 YPELAER, GABRIEL: Affectionis hypochondriacae historiam et curandi modum continens. Leyden 1661 (2).

1081 ZACHLER, J. CHR. – Prof. J. J. STAHL: De immoderato anxio moerore, morbi mortisque autore. Erfurt 1732 (1).

1082 ZECH, JOHANN MICHAEL – Prof. JUSTUS VESTI: Casum passione hysterica laborantis ejusque curationem proponens. Erfurt 1703.

1083 ZEIDLER: De mania. Leipzig 1630.

1084 ZEYS, VALENT.: De melancholia theses. Basel 1600 (1, 13).

1085 ZIEGLER, JOHANN: Casum viri hypochondriaci exhibens. Basel 1697 (1, 13).

1086 ZIEGNER, GE. – Prof. ANDR. OLTOM. GOELICKE: De officio medici circa superstitionem aegrotorum. Frankfurt a. O. 1733.

1087 ZINDEL, NIC.: De morbis ex castitate nimia oriundis. Basel 1745 (1).

1088 ZOPFF, JO. CHR. – Prof. GEORG WOLFGANG WEDEL: De morbo hypochondriaco. Jena 1676 (6, 12).

1089 ZORNIUS, PETER: De philtris enthusiasticis Anglico-Batavicis, oder von dem Englischen und Holländischen Quäcker-Pulver. Rostock 1707 (24).

1090 ZUR MÜHLEN, GERHARDUS – Prof. THEODOR CRAANEN: De melancholia. Leyden 1676 (8).

1091 ZWICKY, CASPAR: De phrenitide. Basel 1706 (1).

1092 ZWINGER, JAC.: De somno eiusque causis et accidentibus cum naturalibus tum praeter naturam. Basel 1594 (1, 8, 13).

1093 ZWINGER, FRIEDRICH: De paraphrenitide. Basel 1731 (1, 8, 12).

1094 ZYL, DOM. VAN: De memoria ejusque vities. Leyden 1694.

Additional Dissertations

1095 Bobin, Gregorius Benjamin: Exhibens compendiosam famosi quod hypochondria vexat. Würzburg 1745 (13).

1096 Harmes, Henr. Ludolph: Diss. in causes morborum et mortis subjecti ejusdam maniaci. Königsberg 1744 (13).

1097 Offredus, Paulus: Quaestiones medicae. Basel 1603 (1, 13).

1098 Reineccius, Johann Paulus: Num Daemon cum sagis generare possit. Wittenberg 1676 (13).

1099 Rey, Guillelmus: De causis delirii in genere. Montpellier 1714 (13).

1100 Steffan, Joh. Jacob: De somnambulis. Basel 1701 (1, 13).

a) Collected Dissertations Printed by the Presiding Professor

Horst, Gregor: Conciliator enucleatus. Giessen 1615, bound with De natura amoris. Giessen 1611.

Horst, Gregor: Disputationum viginti. Wittenberg 1609, bound with Jacob Horst: Disputationes Catholicae de rebus secundum et praeter naturam.

Knoblochius, Tobias: Institutiones anatomicae et psychologicae. Wittenberg 1612, 1661.

Liddel, Duncan: Universae medicinae compendium. Helmstadt 1620.

Rolfinck, Werner: Epitome methodi cognoscendi et curandi adfectus capitis particulares. Jena 1655.

Rolfinck, Werner: Ordus et methodus medicinae specialis. Jena 1669, 1671.

Tandler, Tobias: Dissertationes physicae medicae. 1613.

Waldschmidt, Joh. Jacob: Opera medica practica. Frankfurt a. M. 1695.

Presiding Professors

This list is necessarily incomplete as in many universities the name of the presiding professor was not included in the printed dissertation.

ADOLPHI, CHR. M. 902
AGERIUS, NIC. 390, 459, 875
AIGNAN, FRANC. 904
AKAKIA, M. 73, 587
ALBERTI, M. 48, 49, 190, 332, 334,
    342, 353, 441, 442, 452, 461, 482,
    503, 518, 577, 667, 674, 722, 730,
    738, 768, 859, 888, 960, 967,
    1013, 1030, 1037, 1045, 1048
ALBINUS, B. 15, 554, 637, 638, 699,
    706, 718, 1068
ALBRECHT, JO. W. 731
AMAN, P. 822
ANCHERSON, A. 278, 704, 953
ANDREAE, TOB. 120
ANDREAS, JO. 440
ASTRUC, JO. 669
AURACHER, S. JAC. 34
BAIER, JO. JAC. 739
BAIER, GUILIELMUS 837
BAILLY, N. 349
BANZER, MA. 882
BARNSTOFF, E. 748
BARTHOLINUS, C. 545
BAUHIN, C. 867
BECKHER, DA. 586
BELET, G. 462
BERGER, JO. G. 336, 446, 818
BERNARD, J. J. 340
BLOSSIUS, S. 682
BLUM, M. 938
BOHN, JO. 1058
BORRICHIUS, CL. 115

BOURDELIN, L. CL. 52
BOURGAUD, JO. A. 995
BOURGEOIS, JO. 548
BOYVIN, CL. 72
BRAYER, C. 228
BRENDEL, A. 134
BRENDEL, Z. 891, 935
BRODTBECK, CO. 526
BRUNNER, JO. C. 550
BURCHARDUS, CHR. M. 695
BÜCHNER, A. E. 12, 135, 141, 317,
    431, 892, 947
BÜTTNER, JO. DA. 785
CHLADENIUS, M. 589
CAMERARIUS, AL. 17, 370
CAMERARIUS, EL. 119, 204, 478, 693
CAMERARIUS, EL. R. 8, 331, 1040
CAMERARIUS, R. JA. 124
CARON, PH. 367
CARRÉ, JAC. JUL. 603
CHARSTADIUS, V. 969
CHEMINEAU, A. N. 559
CLAUSING, H. 1067
COCCIUS, JO. 665
COL DE VILARS, ELIA 301
COLIUS, JAC. 829
COLLIER, P. 393
CONRING, H. 121, 226, 411
CORDELLE, JO. 573
CORNUTY, JAC. 114
COSNIER, H. 37
COUSINOT, JAC. 266, 791
CRAANEN, TH. 835